theclinics.com

THORACIC SURGERY CLINICS

Preoperative Evaluation of Lung Resection Candidates

GUEST EDITOR
Alessandro Brunelli, MD

CONSULTING EDITOR
Mark K. Ferguson, MD

February 2008 • Volume 18 • Number 1

SAUNDERS

An Imprint of Elsevier, Inc.
PHILADELPHIA LONDON TORONTO MONTREAL SYDNEY TOKYO

W.B. SAUNDERS COMPANY
A Division of Elsevier Inc.

1600 John F. Kennedy Boulevard, Suite 1800 • Philadelphia, Pennsylvania 19103-2899

http://www.theclinics.com

THORACIC SURGERY CLINICS
February 2008
Editor: Catherine Bewick

Volume 18, Number 1
ISSN 1547-4127
ISBN-13: 978-1-4160-5808-3
ISBN-10: 1-4160-5808-7

Thoracic Surgery Clinics (ISSN 1547-4127) is published quarterly by Elsevier Inc., 360 Park Avenue South, New York, NY 10010-1710. Months of publication are February, May, August, and November. Business and editorial offices: 1600 John F. Kennedy Boulevard, Suite 1800, Philadelphia, PA 19103-2899. Customer service office: 6277 Sea Harbor Drive, Orlando, FL 32887-4800. Periodicals postage paid at New York, NY, and additional mailing offices. Subscription prices are $220.00 per year (US individuals), $321.00 per year (US institutions), $110.00 per year (US students), $281.00 per year (Canadian individuals), $398.00 per year (Canadian institutions), $141.00 per year (Canadian and foreign students), $281.00 per year (foreign individuals), and $398.00 per year (foreign institutions). Foreign air speed delivery is included in all *Clinics'* subscription prices. All prices are subject to change without notice. POSTMASTER: Send address changes to *Thoracic Surgery Clinics*, Elsevier Journals Customer Service, 6277 Sea Harbor Drive, Orlando, FL 32887-4800. **Customer Service: 1-800-654-2452 (US). From outside of the US, call 1-407-563-6020. Fax: 1-407-363-9661.** E-mail: JournalsCustomerService-usa@elsevier.com

Reprints. For copies of 100 or more, of articles in this publication, please contact Commercial Rights Department, Elsevier Inc., 360 Park Avenue South, New York, NY 10010-1710. Tel: (212) 633-3813; Fax: (212) 462-1935; e-mail: reprints@elsevier.com.

Thoracic Surgery Clinics is covered in *Index Medicus* and *EMBASE/Excerpta Medica*.

Printed in the United States of America.

CONSULTING EDITOR

MARK K. FERGUSON, MD, Professor of Surgery, Section of Cardiac and Thoracic Surgery, The University of Chicago, Chicago, Illinois

GUEST EDITOR

ALESSANDRO BRUNELLI, MD, Staff Thoracic Surgeon, Division of Thoracic Surgery, Umberto I Regional Hospital, Ancona, Italy

CONTRIBUTORS

CHRIS T. BOLLIGER, MD, PhD, Director of Respiratory Research and Co-Chairman, Division of Pulmonology, Department of Medicine, Faculty of Health Sciences, University of Stellenbosch, Cape Town, South Africa

ALESSANDRO BRUNELLI, MD, Staff Thoracic Surgeon, Division of Thoracic Surgery, Umberto I Regional Hospital, Ancona, Italy

AYESHA S. BRYANT, MSPH, MD, Assistant Professor, Division of Cardiothoracic Surgery, Department of Surgery, University of Alabama at Birmingham; and Department of Epidemiology, University of Alabama at Birmingham School of Public Health, Birmingham, Alabama

JOHN CANNON, MBBS, MRCP, Respiratory Registrar, Respiratory Medicine, Lister Hospital, Stevenage, United Kingdom

ROBERT J. CERFOLIO, MD, FACS, FCCP, Professor and Chief, Division of Cardiothoracic Surgery, Department of Surgery, University of Alabama at Birmingham, Birmingham, Alabama

STEVEN L. COHN, MD, FACP, Chief, Division of General Internal Medicine; Clinical Professor of Medicine, SUNY Downstate Medical Center; and Director, Medical Consultation Service, Kings County Hospital, Brooklyn, New York

TIMOTHY W. EVANS, MD, PhD, Professor of Intensive Care, Department of Thoracic Surgery, Royal Brompton Hospital; and Department of Intensive Care Medicine, Imperial College School of Medicine, Royal Brompton Hospital, London, United Kingdom

MARK K. FERGUSON, MD, Professor of Surgery, Section of Cardiac and Thoracic Surgery, The University of Chicago, Chicago, Illinois

SIMON JORDAN, MD, FRCS, Consultant Thoracic Surgeon, Department of Thoracic Surgery, Royal Brompton Hospital; and Department of Intensive Care Medicine, Imperial College School of Medicine, Royal Brompton Hospital, London, United Kingdom

COENRAAD F.N. KOEGELENBERG, MBChB, FCP(SA), MRCP(UK), Senior Specialist, Division of Pulmonology, Department of Medicine, Faculty of Health Sciences, University of Stellenbosch, Cape Town, South Africa

RODNEY J. LANDRENEAU, MD, Professor of Surgery, Division of Thoracic and Foregut Surgery, Heart, Lung, and Esophageal Surgery Institute, University of Pittsburgh Medical Center, Pittsburgh, Pennsylvania

AMY G. LEHMAN, MD, MBA, Department of Surgery, The University of Chicago, Chicago, Illinois

JAMES D. LUKETICH, MD, Henry Bahnson Professor of Surgery and Chief, Division of Thoracic and Foregut Surgery, Heart, Lung, and Esophageal Surgery Institute, University of Pittsburgh Medical Center, Pittsburgh, Pennsylvania

LINDA NICI, MD, Clinical Associate Professor of Medicine, Brown University School of Medicine; and Associate Chief, Pulmonary and Critical Care Section, Providence Veterans Administration Medical Center, Providence, Rhode Island

NURIA M. NOVOA, MD, PhD, Service of Thoracic Surgery, Salamanca University Hospital, Salamanca, Spain

BRIAN L. PETTIFORD, MD, Assistant Professor of Surgery, Division of Thoracic and Foregut Surgery, Heart, Lung, and Esophageal Surgery Institute, University of Pittsburgh Medical Center, Pittsburgh, Pennsylvania

GAETANO ROCCO, MD, FRCS, Division of Thoracic Surgery, National Cancer Institute, Pascale Foundation, Naples, Italy

MATTHEW J. SCHUCHERT, MD, Assistant Professor of Surgery, Division of Thoracic and Foregut Surgery, Heart, Lung, and Esophageal Surgery Institute, University of Pittsburgh Medical Center, Pittsburgh, Pennsylvania

GEORGIOS STAMATIS, FETCS, Professor for Surgery, Department of Thoracic Surgery and Endoscopy, Ruhrlandklinik Essen-Heidhausen, Essen, Germany

TOM TREASURE, MD, FRCS, Clinical Operational Research Unit, University College London, London, United Kingdom

MARTIN UTLEY, PhD, Clinical Operational Research Unit, University College London, London, United Kingdom

GONZALO VARELA, MD, PhD, FETCS, Professor of Thoracic Surgery and Head, Service of Thoracic Surgery, Salamanca University Hospital, Salamanca, Spain

THIDA WIN, MD, MRCP, Consultant Physician, Respiratory Medicine, Lister Hospital, Stevenage, United Kingdom

CONTENTS

FORTHCOMING ISSUES

May 2008

Hyperhidrosis
Sean Grondin, MD, *Guest Editor*

August 2008

Minimally Invasive Thoracic Surgery
Gaetano Rocco, MD, FRCS (Ed), FECTS, *Guest Editor*

November 2008

Management of N2/IIIA Lung Cancer
M. Sukumar, *Guest Editor*

RECENT ISSUES

November 2007

Thoracic Anatomy, Part I: Chest Wall, Airway, Lungs
Jean Deslauriers, MD, FRCS(C), *Guest Editor*

August 2007

Risk Prediction and Outcome Analysis in Thoracic Surgery
Gaetano Rocco, MD, FRCS (Ed), FECTS, *Guest Editor*

May 2007

Management of Stage I Non-Small Cell Lung Cancer
Rodney J. Landreneau, MD, *Guest Editor*

ELSEVIER
SAUNDERS

Thorac Surg Clin 18 (2008) xi

THORACIC
SURGERY
CLINICS

Preface

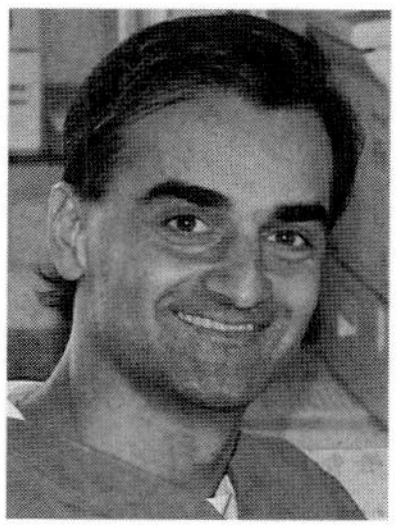

Alessandro Brunelli, MD
Guest Editor

Thoracic surgeons are faced with an increasing population of elderly patients who have underlying multiple comorbidities and who have an increased risk of postoperative morbidity and mortality. In addition, managed care systems demand an increased effort in delivering high standards of quality of care in a context of cost-containment. This challenging scenario can only be coped with by optimizing clinical pathways of care.

In this regard, the preoperative evaluation of candidates for lung resection may serve multiple purposes: minimize the improper exclusion of patients from operation; optimize the perioperative treatment with the aim to reduce postoperative complications; plan a postoperative advanced care management; select, whenever oncologically and technically feasible, the extent of the resection; and obtain a more informed consent from the patient. Furthermore, an accurate preoperative risk-stratification may be used for audit purposes and for a more accurate allocation of institutional resources.

In this issue of *Thoracic Surgery Clinics*, the preoperative evaluation of the lung resection candidate has been put into perspective regarding important issues, such as the declining role of predicted postoperative forced expiratory volume in one second in favor of more global tests of fitness (exercise tests), the accuracy of split lung function assessment, the importance of preoperative and postoperative cardiopulmonary rehabilitation, the need for postoperative intensive care unit management, current trends in cardiac evaluation and cardiac risk assessment—particularly in light of the increasing number of patients presenting with concomitant coronary artery disease the risk of the ever-increasing multimodality approach to lung cancer patients, the role of limited resections in compromised patients, the residual quality of life after lung resection, the controversial use of risk-models for patients selection, the application of risk-stratification in assisting perioperative fast-tracking, and a glimpse into the future of preoperative functional evaluation.

Experts in the field have contributed to enlighten readers about these often controversial topics, which are so important for the practicing thoracic surgeon.

Alessandro Brunelli, MD
Division of Thoracic Surgery
Umberto I Regional Hospital
Via Conca 1
60020 Torrette
Ancona, Italy

E-mail address: Alexit_2000@yahoo.com

doi:10.1016/j.thorsurg.2007.11.002

ELSEVIER
SAUNDERS

Thorac Surg Clin 18 (2008) 1–8

THORACIC
SURGERY
CLINICS

Spirometry: Predicting Risk and Outcome

Alessandro Brunelli, MD[a,*], Gaetano Rocco, MD, FRCS[a,b]

[a]*Unit of Thoracic Surgery, Umberto I Regional Hospital, Via Conca 1, 60020 Torrette, Ancona 60124, Italy*
[b]*Division of Thoracic Surgery, National Cancer Institute, Pascale Foundation, Via Semmola 81, 80131 Naples, Italy*

Interest in identifying patients at risk for postoperative pulmonary complications came from early surgical observations [1] that this class of complications was the most frequent cause of morbidity and mortality in the postoperative period. Simple tests of pulmonary function were sought as ways of defining surgical risk. In the 1950s, several investigators confirmed that abnormalities in timed segments of spirometric tracing, analyzed in conjunction with forced vital capacity, identified patients who would suffer pulmonary disability or mortality after thoracic surgery [2–5]. The ease of doing spirometric evaluation in ill patients, coupled with technical advances, resulted in rapid proliferation of this technology. Based on these studies, it was concluded that pulmonary function testing was more sensitive than history and physical examination for detecting lung disease and for predicting postoperative complications. An anecdote may well explain the context of risk prediction in earlier days. Not many years ago, during a busy afternoon dedicated to an outpatient clinic in the residency years, the trainee was evaluating a patient with both lung cancer and what he perceived as a terrible pulmonary reserve. With the spirometry sheet firm in one hand and the computerized tomographic scan of the chest in the other, the resident raced next door where his mentor, a world famous thoracic surgeon, was also seeing patients for the following day operative list. The resident must have had a startled expression—almost feeling insulted that a pulmonologist would have dared propose such a patient for surgery. The mentor glanced for a short second at the documentation then a few wrinkles flattened on his forehead and whispered: "If he can talk, he can have an operation!"

Clinical instinct has always been the main driving intellectual force in the preoperative assessment of candidates to lung surgery. The more the surgeon's expertise and experience grew in the developments of his or her career, the further from emphasizing the results of preoperative investigations in the evaluation he or she would be. The advent of the concept of evidence-based medicine (and surgery), the sky-rocketing advancements in anesthesiology and treatment of end-stage pulmonary failure (culminating in lung transplantation), and the intolerable levels of medico-legal litigation have all contributed to leaving surgeons having to rely on numbers to support their clinical decisions. In addition, the publication of manuscripts focused on the patients' perception of surgical outcome has made surgeons increasingly aware that their idea of outcome may not necessarily coincide with the one shared by their patients.

The fact that matters is that in 2007 thoracic surgeons are still performing pulmonary resections, with mortality rates at best doubled when compared with by-pass coronary artery grafting [6,7]. Mortality and morbidity rates are still high when the removal of the entire lung is required—unacceptably high for some who, rightfully so, define pneumonectomy "a disease of its own" [8]. There is a kind of unspoken consensus within the international thoracic surgical community on the fact that surgeons are about to reach the peak of current technical refinement, by extending the use of parenchyma-sparing resections and video-assisted thoracic surgery and introducing robotically guided surgery. Likewise, surgeons are

* Corresponding author.
E-mail address: alexit_2000@yahoo.com
(A. Brunelli).

1547-4127/08/$ - see front matter
doi:10.1016/j.thorsurg.2007.10.007

thoracic.theclinics.com

understanding that to abate morbidity and mortality rates, they need to identify risk factors that are predominantly respiratory, without neglecting the importance of the comorbidities.

The evolution of the risk assessment process has focused on a recurring argumentation, that is the need for guidelines and score systems to objectify the "defective" individual discriminating ability. In this setting, some questions have been raised and tentatively answered: First, is forced expiratory volume (FEV_1) the only predictor for morbidity and mortality? And second, are there alternative predictive factors?

For decades, surgery has been the mainstay of treatment in early stage lung cancer as well as complex infectious conditions of the lung. Concomitantly, FEV_1 alone has been the discriminating parameter of surgical eligibility, as demonstrated by recently published series [9,10]. However, the limitations of FEV_1 emerged in the literature inasmuch as it could lead to the inappropriate exclusion from a surgical option for patients with apparently marginal respiratory function [11] and could not reliably be related to the overall surgical outcome or the patient's perception of this outcome [12,13]. Carbon monoxide diffusing capacity (DLCO) was then suggested as a complementary parameter to be introduced along with the concept of defining numeric values corresponding to the predicted postoperative (ppo) figures of FEV_1 and DLCO [14–16]. Currently available and widely applied guidelines, devised by the American College of Chest Physicians (ACCP) and the British Thoracic Society (BTS), revolve around this FEV_1-centered, DLCO-confirmed evaluation of the candidates to lung resection [6,17]. However, recent evidence argues against the predicting ability of $ppoFEV_1$ and ppoDLCO, especially in the immediate postoperative period and in patients with severe airflow limitation [18,19], emphasizing the predictive potential for major morbidity of the "worst case" FEV_1: that is, the FEV_1 measured immediately after surgery.

Current functional algorithms using pulmonary function tests

The two most commonly used algorithms for the preoperative evaluation of the cardiorespiratory function of candidates for lung resection are those published on behalf of the BTS and ACCP [6,17].

The BTS guidelines recommend that all patients with a preoperative FEV_1 greater than 2 liters (L) may undergo up to pneumonectomy, whereas those with a preoperative FEV_1 greater than 1.5 L may undergo up to lobectomy. These recommendations were based on data from more than 2,000 patients in three large series in the 1970s, which showed that a mortality rate of under 5% should be expected if the preoperative FEV_1 is greater than 1.5 L for a lobectomy and greater than 2 L for a pneumonectomy [20–22]. Unfortunately, these studies did not report the percentage of predicted FEV_1, and the values were expressed as absolute numbers, which do not take into account the gender and size of the patients. Absolute values may bias against older patients, people of small stature, and female patients, who might tolerate lower levels of lung function. For those patients with a preoperative FEV_1 below 1.5 L to 2 L, estimation of carbon monoxide lung diffusion capacity is recommended. Furthermore, quantitative lung perfusion scan should be performed to calculate the $ppoFEV_1$ and ppoDLCO.

In the cases of patients with $ppoFEV_1$ and ppoDLCO above 40% of prediction, no further tests are required before the planned resection and patients are considered to have an average operative risk. On the other hand, for those patients with both $ppoFEV_1$ and ppoDLCO lower than 40%, a less extensive resection should be considered whenever possible, or radical radiotherapy, for they are regarded as high-risk patients. Any other combination of $ppoFEV_1$ and ppoDLCO should perform an exercise test. Shuttle walk testing is recommended as first line low-tech exercise. Those patients that walk less than 25 shuttles or are desaturated more than 4% should be regarded as high-risk patients. For all the other patients, a full cardiopulmonary exercise test is recommended, and for those candidates achieving a maximum oxygen consumption (VO_2max) less than 15 mL/kg per minute, nonsurgical options should be considered.

The ACCP guidelines recommend similar FEV_1 criteria for lobectomy and pneumonectomy. For those patients with a preoperative FEV_1 less than 1.5 L to 2 L, or 80%, predicted postoperative lung function should be calculated (by lung perfusion scan for pneumonectomy candidates and by anatomic segmental method for all other lung resections). Patients with $ppoFEV_1$ less than 30% or a predicted postoperative product ($ppoFEV_1$ times ppoDLCO) less than 1,650 are deemed inoperable.

In cases of patients with $ppoFEV_1$ or ppoDLCO less than 40%, a cardiopulmonary exercise test is recommended. If the VO_2max result is less than 10 mL/kg per minute, or in case of VO_2max lower than 15 mL/kg per minute associated with a ppoFEV_1 and ppoDLCO less than 40%, the surgical risk is considered prohibitive.

The role of predicted postoperative forced expiratory volume in risk-stratification before surgery

Many studies have shown the role of ppo$FEV_1$1 in predicting postoperative complications and in selecting patients for surgery. Olsen and colleagues [23] suggested a threshold value of 0.8 L as the lower limit for surgical resection. However, Pate and colleagues [24] found that patients with a mean ppoFEV_1 of 0.7 L tolerated thoracotomy for lung cancer resection. This experience might have reflected resection of less lung tissue than anticipated. Again the main objection to using an absolute value of ppoFEV_1 as a threshold for operability is that it might prevent older patients, small stature people, and females patients, all of whom might tolerate a lower absolute FEV_1, from having a potentially curative lung cancer resection. Consequently, establishing a threshold for lung function expressed as percent ppo (%ppo) rather than absolute ppo would be desirable. Case series with small numbers of patients have shown that perioperative risks increase substantially when the %ppoFEV_1 is less than 40% of predicted normal [15,16,25–28].

Markos and colleagues [15] reported that three out of six patients with a %ppoFEV_1 less than 40% died in the perioperative period. Wahi and colleagues [28] found a perioperative mortality rate of 16% in patients with a %ppo FEV_1 of less than 41%, versus 3% among those with better predicted lung function. Pierce and colleagues [16] found that five out of thirteen patients with a %ppoFEV_1 less than 40% died soon after operation, and Bolliger and colleagues [25] reported that two out of four patients with similar lung function died of respiratory failure perioperatively. Similarly, Nakahara and colleagues [29] found an especially high postoperative mortality rate (6 out of 10 patients, 60%) when the %ppoFEV_1 was less than 30%.

Kearney and colleagues [30] found that in 331 patients undergoing lung resection, ppoFEV_1 was the best predictor of complications after controlling the effect of other risk factors in a multivariate analysis. In particular, the incidence of respiratory complications was fivefold higher in patients with ppoFEV_1 less than 1 L, compared with those with a ppoFEV_1 greater than 1.4 L (15% versus 3%, respectively). The total morbidity rate was 34% in patients with a ppoFEV_1 less than 1 L versus 11% in those with ppoFEV_1 greater than 1.4 L.

Ferguson and colleagues [14] were the first to observe that a low ppoDLCO, was a strong predictor of mortality. Subsequently, others have also found that perioperative risks increase substantially when the ppoDLCO is lower than 40% [15,16].

Pierce and colleagues [16] suggested that a product of %ppo FEV_1 and %ppoDLCO less than 1,650 might serve as a more discriminating threshold for perioperative risk assessment. Subsequently, others have made a similar observation [31].

Although ppoFEV_1 and ppoDLCO less than 40% indicate increased risk for perioperative complications and mortality from lung cancer resection, Ribas and colleagues [31] showed that these patients can be successfully operated on. They described a selected group of 65 patients who met these physiologic criteria but still underwent curative intent lobectomy and wedge resections (n = 44) or pneumonectomies (n = 21). There were only four postoperative deaths (6.2% mortality rate), and cardiopulmonary complications occurred in 31 patients (47.7%). This study is important because it indicates that predictive postoperative pulmonary function cannot be used alone to screen patients for surgery, and that more sophisticated tests are needed—especially in high risk patients—for determining their suitability for pulmonary resection.

The role of DLCO in predicting complications after lung resection has led to the incorporation of this measurement in functional algorithms in selected patients with impaired pulmonary function (FEV_1 less than 80% of predicted) (ACCP, BTS). However, the approach to select patients for DLCO testing based on their FEV_1 values should be warranted only in case of a high correlation between these two variables. Because FEV_1 and DLCO reflect the status of two different components of the pulmonary function (airflow and gas exchange), they may not be necessarily correlated between each other. In a recent study from Brunelli and colleagues [32] analyzing 872 patients submitted to lung resection after systematic preoperative measurement of DLCO, diffusion resulted modestly correlated with FEV_1 in the entire population and in groups of patients stratified by age, gender, cause of operation, and airflow limitation. In particular, 43% of patients with FEV_1 greater than 80% had DLCO less than 80%, and 24% of them had a DLCO less than 70%. In this group of patients without airflow limitation, logistic regression showed that a ppoDLCO less than 40% was a significant and reliable predictor of postoperative cardiopulmonary complications. The investigators concluded that the approach to select patients for DLCO measurement based on their degree of airflow limitation is not justified, given the only modest correlation between FEV_1 and DLCO in these patients. Based on their results, they recommended the routine measurement of DLCO in all candidates for lung resection, irrespective of their FEV_1 value, to improve surgical risk stratification.

Predicted postoperative forced expiratory volume in patients with chronic obstructive pulmonary disease

PpoFEV1 is pivotal in the two most widely used functional algorithms for evaluating patients before lung resection. In certain circumstances, this parameter is used alone to include or even exclude patients from operation without further evaluations. However, a recent paper from Brunelli and colleagues [19] showed that whereas $ppoFEV_1$ was the only significant predictor of cardiopulmonary complications in 450 patients without airflow limitations (FEV_1 greater than 70%) submitted to major lung resection, in those patients with FEV_1 less than 70% (94 patients) $ppoFEV_1$ was not a reliable predictor of complications. Furthermore, in those patients with a $ppoFEV_1$ less than 40%, the morbidity and mortality rates were only 28.6% and 4.8%, respectively. These findings may be partly explained by the so-called "lung volume reduction effect" that can reduce the functional loss in patients with airflow limitations. In candidates for lobectomy with lung cancer and moderate to severe chronic obstructive pulmonary disease (COPD), the resection of the most affected parenchyma may determine an actual improvement in the elastic recoil, a reduction of the airflow resistance, and an improvement in pulmonary mechanics and V/Q matching, similar to what happens in typical candidates for lung volume reduction surgery with end-stage hetherogeneous emphysema [33,34]. In this regard, many studies have already shown the minimal loss or even the improvement in pulmonary function after lobectomy in these obstructed patients, questioning the traditional operability criteria mostly based on pulmonary parameters.

Korst and colleagues [35] showed that in a group of 13 patients with preoperative FEV_1 less than 60%, and FEV_1 to forced vital capacity (FVC) ratio less than 0.6, the FEV_1 improved 4% 4 months after lobectomy. In the group of patients with FEV_1 less than 80% but greater than 60% (median 69%), the FEV_1 measured at 4 months after lobectomy was 16% lower than the preoperative value. These investigators defined a COPD index to characterize the purity of COPD (FEV_1-percent of predicted in decimal form plus FEV_1/FVC ratio). They found that as the preoperative COPD-index fell below 1 (implying more severe and pure COPD), the more likely it was that FEV_1 increased after lobectomy.

Carretta and colleagues [36] reported an FEV_1 improvement of 5% and an airway resistance decrease of 27% in the 10 patients with higher degree of obstruction 2 to 7 months after operation. On the other hand, in the group of patients with a less severe degree of obstruction, the FEV_1 decreased 6%.

Santambrogio and colleagues [37] showed that, whereas non-COPD patients had a mean reduction in FEV_1 of 15% 6 months after lobectomy, those patients with preoperative FEV_1 less than 80% had a minimal loss of only 3%. Among these patients, the subgroup with the highest degree of obstruction (FEV_1 between 40% and 64%) had an increase in their FEV_1 of 3.4%, compared with preoperative values. The investigators also found that preoperative FEV_1 was the only independent factor associated with the postoperative change in FEV_1 in a multivariate regression analysis.

Edwards and colleagues [38] divided 29 patients with emphysema in two groups according to their $ppoFEV_1$ above or below 40%. In those patients with a $ppoFEV_1$ less than 40%, no difference was noted between preoperative and postoperative FEV_1, as assessed 3 months after the operation. Moreover, in this group the actual postoperative FEV_1 3 months after the operation was 10% higher than predicted (41.5% versus 31%). In the other group, those with a $ppoFEV_1$ greater than 40%, the postoperative FEV_1 was 25% lower than the preoperative value, and no difference was noted between predicted and observed postoperative FEV_1 (47.3% versus 46.6%).

Sekine and colleagues [39] followed 48 patients with FEV_1 less than 70% and FEV_1/FVC ratio less than 0.7. They found an actual to predicted postoperative FEV_1 ratio of 1.1 in COPD patients

1 month after surgery, versus 0.9 in the 473 non-COPD patients. The FEV_1 loss in COPD patients was only 13%, versus a loss of 29% in non-COPD patients. In this study, COPD and the pulmonary resection of the lower portion of the lung were found to be independent factors for the minimal deterioration (defined as an actual to predicted postoperative FEV_1 ratio of 1.15 or more) of postoperative FEV_1 in a logistic regression analysis.

In a recent study of Baldi and colleagues [40], 88 COPD patients were analyzed before and within 6 months after operation. In those patients with FEV_1 less than 80% the actual to predicted postoperative, FEV_1 was 1.21. In these patients the observed postoperative FEV_1 value was similar to the preoperative one (65% versus 63%, respectively).

In a recent study, Brunelli and colleagues [41] showed that COPD patients (FEV_1 less than 80% plus FEV_1/FVC ratio less than 0.7) had significantly lower losses of FEV_1 and DLCO, compared with non-COPD patients 3 months after lobectomy for lung cancer (8% versus 16% and 3% versus 12%, respectively). Furthermore, their exercise tolerance, evaluated by a stair-climbing test, was similar to the one observed in non-COPD patients with a calculated VO_2 peak which returned to baseline preoperative values. In this series, 27% of COPD patients actually improved their FEV_1, 34% their DLCO, and 43% their VO_2max 3 months after operation.

In another article, Brunelli and colleagues [42] found that the actual to predicted postoperative (apo/ppo) FEV_1 ratio in COPD patients was 1.11 and 1.15 1 month and 3 months after lobectomy, respectively. They also found that, not only FEV_1 but also DLCO was better than predicted after lobectomy in COPD patients: the apo/ppo DLCO ratios were 1.09 and 1.22 1 month and 3 months after lobectomy, respectively.

The same investigators [43] demonstrated that this lung volume reduction effect may take place very early after lung resection. In a group of 161 patients evaluated at discharge (median 8 days) after lobectomy, they found that in patients with a preoperative FEV_1 less than 70%, the mean FEV_1 loss was only 12.6%, versus a mean loss of 30% in those with FEV_1 greater than 70%. Seventeen percent of the obstructed patients actually improved their FEV_1 at discharge.

This early lung volume reduction effect was confirmed by Varela and colleagues [44], who showed that the percentage loss of FEV_1 measured on the first postoperative day after lobectomy was lower in patients with lower COPD-index, a parameter inversely correlated with the degree and purity of obstructive disease.

These findings show that ppoFEV_1 may not work properly in those patients with obstructive disease, and cannot be used alone to select patients for operation, especially those with limited pulmonary functions.

Predicted postoperative forced expiratory volume and observed forced expiratory volume in the first postoperative days

Although many studies have shown that ppo-FEV_1 is fairly accurate in predicting the definitive residual FEV_1 3 to 6 months after surgery [15,23,41,45–51], it has been recently demonstrated that it substantially overestimates the actual FEV_1 observed in the first postoperative days, when most of the complications occur [52].

A prospective consecutive series of 125 uneventful lobectomy patients were analyzed by serial measurements of FEV_1 preoperatively and during the 6 postoperative days until discharge by a portable spirometer. The mean FEV_1 on postoperative day 1 was 47%, and increased up to 58.6% on postoperative day 6 (plus 25%). Despite this increase, the postoperative FEV_1 never reached the ppoFEV_1 value. In fact, on postoperative day 1 the actual to predicted FEV_1 ratio was 0.71 and reached 0.93 on postoperative day 6. The investigators showed that the actual FEV_1 on the first postoperative day is about 30% lower than predicted. This may have serious clinical implications whenever using ppoFEV_1 for patient selection and risk-stratification before operation.

A time-series cross-sectional regression analysis was also performed to assess the factors associated with the changes in FEV_1 ratio during the postoperative period. The investigators found that factors reliably associated with apo/ppo FEV_1 ratio were preoperative FEV_1 value (lower preoperative FEV_1, higher postoperative FEV_1 ratio), pain score (higher score, lower FEV_1 ratio), and the presence of epidural analgesia. These results highlighted the importance of an adequate pain control in the early postoperative phase and the early effect of the lung volume reduction effect in patients with preoperative lower FEV_1 values undergoing lobectomy. Certainly, current methods of prediction of the postoperative FEV_1 greatly underestimate the functional loss in the early postoperative phase. Therefore, for the purpose of a more accurate risk stratification, investigators may need to correct the traditional prediction of postoperative FEV_1.

This concept was further corroborated by the results of a recently published analysis on the role of first-day FEV_1 in predicting cardiorespiratory complications after major lung resection. In a prospective series of 198 major lung resections, Varela and colleagues [18] demonstrated, through a classification tree analysis that the FEV_1 measured the first postoperative day was a better predictor of complications when compared with ppoFEV_1 (100% versus 43% importance as primary splitter or surrogate of other variables, respectively). Probably the predictive value of ppoFEV_1 assigned by several investigators is a result of the correlation existing between ppoFEV_1 and first-day FEV_1 ($r = 0.56$, $P < .01$).

Prompted by the results of these studies, Brunelli and colleagues [53] developed and validated a model to estimate the value of FEV_1 on the first postoperative day after major lung resection. Factors reliably associated with postoperative first-day FEV_1 were age ($P = .002$), preoperative FEV_1 ($P < .0001$), the presence of epidural analgesia ($P < .0001$), and the percentage of nonobstructed segments removed during operation ($P = .001$). The following model estimating the first-day postoperative FEV_1 was derived: $-2.648 + 0.295 \times \text{age} + 0.371 \times FEV_1 + 8.216 \times \text{epidural analgesia} - 0.338 \times \text{percentage of nonobstructed segments removed during operation}$. In an external validation set, the mean predicted first-day postoperative FEV_1 value did not differ from the observed one (42.6 versus 42.0, respectively; $P = .3$) and the plot of the observed versus the predicted first-day FEV_1 showed a satisfactory calibration. If future analyses will prove its role in stratifying the early postoperative risk, this newly developed model may be integrated in preoperative evaluation algorithms to refine risk-stratification.

Summary

Predicted postoperative FEV_1 is certainly the most widely used parameter in preoperative risk stratification [54] and the measure recommend by BTS and ACCP functional guidelines as a first step in the screening of patients for lung resection surgery.

Nevertheless, recent evidences have demonstrated that ppoFEV_1 is not a reliable predictor of postoperative cardiopulmonary complications in patients with preoperative impaired pulmonary function. This may be because of the fact that the resection of a portion of lung in patients with obstructive disease determines only a minimal loss, or even an improvement, in overall respiratory function and exercise tolerance. This lung volume reduction effect takes place very early, since the first postoperative days, balancing what ever negative physiologic effects a thoracotomy and lung resection may entail. In addition to its poor predictive role in COPD patients, ppoFEV_1 largely underestimate the actual loss in the very first days after operation, when most of the complications develop. The rationale to use a parameter which is poorly correlated with the pulmonary function at the moment the complications occur seems unwarranted. At the very best, ppoFEV_1 appears a weak surrogate of the immediate postoperative FEV_1. The FEV_1 measured on the first postoperative day may be 30% less than predicted. Corrective equations have been published to correct this discrepancy with the aim to improve risk stratification.

References

[1] King DS. Postoperative pulmonary complications: a statistical study based on two years' personal observation. Surg Gynecol Obstet 1932;56:43–50.
[2] Gaensler EA, Cugell DW, Lindgren I, et al. The role of pulmonary insufficiency in mortality and invalidism following surgery for pulmonary tuberculosis. J Thorac Cardiovasc Surg 1955;29:163–87.
[3] Miller WF, Wu N, Johnson RL Jr. Convenient method for evaluating pulmonary ventilatory function with a single breath test. Anesthesiology 1956;17:480–93.
[4] Gaensler EA. Analysis of the ventilatory defect by timed capacity measurements. Am Rev Tuberc 1951;64:256–78.
[5] Woodruff W, Merkel CG, Wright GW. Decision in thoracic surgery as influenced by the knowledge of pulmonary physiology. J Thorac Surg 1953;26:156–83.
[6] British Thoracic Society; Society of Cardiothoracic Surgeons of Great Britain and Ireland Working Party. BTS Guidelines: guidelines on the selection of patients with lung cancer for surgery. Thorax 2001;56:89–108.
[7] Society for Cardiothoracic Surgery in Great Britian and Ireland. Audits and outcomes. Available at: http://wwwscts.org/sections/audit/index.html. Accessed October 25, 2007.
[8] Deslauriers J. Invited commentary. Ann Thorac Surg 2001;72:1154.
[9] Licker MJ, Widikker I, Robert J, et al. Operative mortality and respiratory complications after lung resection for cancer: impact of chronic obstructive

pulmonary disease and time trends. Ann Thorac Surg 2006;81:1830–7.

[10] Rocco G. Invited commentary. Ann Thorac Surg 2006;81:1837–8.

[11] Linden PA, Bueno R, Colson YL, et al. Lung resection in patients with preoperative FEV1 < 35% predicted. Chest 2005;127:1984–90.

[12] Sekine Y, Kelser KA, Behnia M, et al. COPD may increase the incidence of refractory supraventricular arrhythmias following pulmonary resection for non small cell lung cancer. Chest 2001;120:1783–90.

[13] Rocco G. Predicting the postoperative outcome after lung surgery. Chest 2001;120:1761.

[14] Ferguson MK, Little L, Rizzo L, et al. Diffusing capacity predicts morbidity and mortality after pulmonary resection. J Thorac Cardiovasc Surg 1988;96:894–900.

[15] Markos J, Mullan BP, Hillman DR, et al. Preoperative assessment as a predictor of mortality and morbidity after lung resection. Am Rev Respir Dis 1989;139:902–10.

[16] Pierce RJ, Copland JM, Sharpe K, et al. Preoperative risk evaluation for lung cancer resection: predicted postoperative product as a predictor of surgical mortality. Am J Respir Crit Care Med 1994;150:947–55.

[17] Colice GL, Shafazand S, Griffin JP, et al. Physiologic evaluation of the patient with lung cancer being considered for resectional surgery. ACCP Evidenced-Based Clinical Practice Guidelines (2nd edition). Chest 2007;132:161S–77S.

[18] Varela G, Brunelli A, Rocco R, et al. Measured FEV1 in the first postoperative day and not ppoFEV1, is the best predictor of cardio-respiratory morbidity after lung resection. Eur J Cardiothorac Surg 2007;31:518–21.

[19] Brunelli A, Al Refai M, Monteverde M, et al. Predictors of early morbidity after major lung resection in patients with and without airflow limitation. Ann Thorac Surg 2002;74:999–1003.

[20] Boushy SF, Billig DM, North LB, et al. Clinical course related to preoperative and postoperative pulmonary function in patients with bronchogenic carcinoma. Chest 1971;59:383–91.

[21] Wernly JA, DeMeester TR, Kirchner PT, et al. Clinical value of quantitative ventilation-perfusion lung scans in the surgical management of bronchogenic carcinoma. J Thorac Cardiovasc Surg 1980;80:535–43.

[22] Miller JI. Physiologic evaluation of pulmonary function in the candidate for lung resection. J Thorac Cardiovasc Surg 1993;105:347–52.

[23] Olsen GN, Block AJ, Tobias JA. Prediction of postpneumonectomy pulmonary function using quantitative macroaggregate lung scanning. Chest 1974;66:13–6.

[24] Pate P, Tenholder MF, Griffin JP, et al. Preoperative assessment of the high-risk patient for lung resection. Ann Thorac Surg 1996;61:1494–500.

[25] Bolliger CT, Wyser C, Roser H, et al. Lung scanning and exercise testing for the prediction of postoperative performance in lung resection candidates at increased risk for complications. Chest 1995;108:341–8.

[26] Holden DA, Rice TW, Stelmach K, et al. Exercise testing, 6-min walk, and stair climb in the evaluation of patients at high risk for pulmonary resection. Chest 1992;102:1774–9.

[27] Gass GD, Olsen GN. Preoperative pulmonary function testing to predict postoperative morbidity and mortality. Chest 1986;89:127–35.

[28] Wahi R, McMurtry MJ, DeCaro LF, et al. Determinants of perioperative morbidity and mortality after pneumonectomy. Ann Thorac Surg 1989;48:33–7.

[29] Nakahara K, Ohno K, Hashimoto J, et al. Prediction of postoperative respiratory failure in patients undergoing lung resection for lung cancer. Ann Thorac Surg 1988;46:549–52.

[30] Kearney DJ, Lee TH, Reilly JJ, et al. Assessment of operative risk in patients undergoing lung resection. Importance of predicted pulmonary function. Chest 1994;105:753–9.

[31] Ribas J, Diaz O, Barbera JA, et al. Invasive exercise testing in the evaluation of patients at high-risk for lung resection. Eur Respir J 1998;12:1429–35

[32] Brunelli A, Refai M, Salati M, et al. Carbon monoxide lung diffusion capacity improves risk-stratification in patients without airflow limitation: evidence for systematic measurement before lung resection. Eur J Cardiothorac Surg 2006;29:567–70.

[33] Cooper JD, Trulock EP, Triantafillou AN, et al. Bilateral pneumectomy (volume reduction) for chronic obstructive pulmonary disease. J Thorac Cardiovasc Surg 1995;109:106–16 [discussion: 116–19].

[34] Ramsey SD, Berry K, Etzioni R, et al. National Emphysema Treatment Trial Research Group. Cost effectiveness of lung-volume-reduction surgery for patients with severe emphysema. N Engl J Med 2003;348:2092–102.

[35] Korst RJ, Ginsberg RJ, Ailawadi M, et al. Lobectomy improves ventilatory function in selected patients with severe COPD. Ann Thorac Surg 1998;66:898–902.

[36] Carretta A, Zannini P, Puglisi A, et al. Improvement of pulmonary function after lobectomy for non-small cell lung cancer in emphysematous patients. Eur J Cardiothorac Surg 1999;15:602–7.

[37] Santambrogio L, Nosotti M, Baisi A, et al. Pulmonary lobectomy for lung cancer: a prospective study to compare patients with forced expiratory volume in 1 s more or less than 80% of predicted. Eur J Cardiothorac Surg 2001;20:684–7.

[38] Edwards JG, Duthie DJ, Waller DA. Lobar volume reduction surgery: a method for increasing the lung cancer resection rate in patients with emphysema. Thorax 2001;56:791–5.

[39] Sekine Y, Iwata T, Chiyo M, et al. Minimal alteration of pulmonary function after lobectomy in lung

cancer patients with chronic obstructive pulmonary disease. Ann Thorac Surg 2003;76:356–61.

[40] Baldi S, Ruffini E, Harari S, et al. Does lobectomy for lung cancer in patients with chronic obstructive pulmonary disease affect lung function? A multicenter national study. J Thorac Cardiovasc Surg 2005; 130:1616–22.

[41] Brunelli A, Refai M, Xiumé F, et al. Evaluation of expiratory volume, diffusion capacity and exercise tolerance following major lung resection: a prospective follow-up analysis. Chest 2007;131:141–7.

[42] Brunelli A, Refai M, Salati M, et al. Predicted versus observed FEV1 and DLCO following major lung resection: a prospective evaluation at different postoperative times. Ann Thorac Surg 2007;83:1134–9.

[43] Brunelli A, Sabbatini A, Xiumé F, et al. A model to predict the decline of the forced expiratory volume in one second and the carbon monoxide lung diffusion capacity early after major lung resection. Interact Cardiovasc Thorac Surg 2005;4:61–5.

[44] Varela G, Brunelli A, Rocco G, et al. Evidence of lower alteration of expiratory volume in patients with airflow limitation in the immediate period after lobectomy. Ann Thorac Surg 2007;84:417–22.

[45] Berend N, Woolcock AJ, Marlin GE. Effects of lobectomy on lung function. Thorax 1980;35:145–50.

[46] Ali MK, Ewer MS, Atallah MR, et al. Regional and overall pulmonary function changes in lung cancer. J Thorac Cardiovasc Surg 1983;86:1–8.

[47] Nakahara K, Monden Y, Ohno K, et al. A method for predicting postoperative lung function and its relation to postoperative complications in patients with lung cancer. Ann Thorac Surg 1985; 39:260–5.

[48] Le Roy Ladurie M, Ranson-Bitker B. Uncertainties in the expected value for forced expiratory volume in one second after surgery. Chest 1986;90:222–8.

[49 Corris PA, Ellis DA, Hawkins T, et al. Use of radionuclide scanning in the preoperative estimation of pulmonary function after pneumonectomy. Thorax 1987;42:285–91.

[50] Pelletier C, Lapointe L, LeBlanc P. Effects of lung resection on pulmonary function and exercise capacity. Thorax 1990;45:497–502.

[51] Bolliger CT, Jordan P, Soler M, et al. Pulmonary function and exercise capacity after lung resection. Eur Respir J 1996;9:415–21.

[52] Varela G, Brunelli A, Rocco G, et al. Predicted versus observed FEV1 in the immediate postoperative period after pulmonary lobectomy. Eur J Cardiothorac Surg 2006;30:644–8.

[53] Brunelli A, Varela G, Rocco G, et al. A model to predict the immediate postoperative FEV1 following major lung resections. Eur J Cardiothorac Surg 2007;32:783–6.

[54] Birim O, Kappetein AP, van Klaveren RJ, et al. Prognostic factors in non-small cell lung cancer surgery. Eur J Surg Oncol 2006;32:12–23.

ELSEVIER
SAUNDERS

Thorac Surg Clin 18 (2008) 9–17

THORACIC
SURGERY
CLINICS

The Role of Diffusing Capacity and Exercise Tests

Mark K. Ferguson, MD[a], Amy G. Lehman, MD, MBA[a], Chris T. Bolliger, MD, PhD[b], Alessandro Brunelli, MD[c,*]

[a]*Department of Surgery, The University of Chicago, 5801 S Ellis Avenue, Chicago, IL 60637, USA*
[b]*Department of Medicine, Division of Pulmonology, Faculty of Health Sciences, University of Stellenbosch, Francie van Zyl Drive, Health Sciences Complex, Tygerberg, 7505, Cape Town, South Africa*
[c]*Unit of Thoracic Surgery, Umberto I Regional Hospital, Via Santa Margherita 23, 60129, Ancona, Italy*

All surgeons who operate on patients with pulmonary malignancies are faced with the daunting task of balancing an individual's preoperative risks with providing effective surgical therapy for the cancer. Risks arise from numerous factors that have been recognized for decades, including comorbidities such as advanced age, cardiovascular disease, poor performance status, and poor pulmonary function. Preoperative pulmonary function testing evaluation grew into more common practice in the 1950s and 1960s, as the frequency of lung resection increased, largely owing to the technical ability to safely perform major lung resection and the rising incidence of lung cancer. Such testing was used to anticipate, and optimally decrease, the incidence of postoperative morbidity and mortality, which were often pulmonary in nature. Such problems include prolonged postoperative mechanical ventilation, other respiratory insufficiency, lobar atelectasis, and pneumonia.

Pulmonary function assessment for the past 50 years has included measurement of arterial blood gases to determine hypoxia or hypercarbia, and pulmonary spirometry, both of which have provided quantitative data to accompany the general clinical evaluation of patients. The utility of spirometric measurements is outlined in "Spirometry: predicting risk and outcomes" by Brunelli and Rocco elsewhere in this issue. Such evaluation, while detailed and relatively objective, has not yielded adequate predictive power of complications after major lung resection. Kooman and colleagues [1] were able to predict only 12% of mortality after pulmonary resection, stating that the remaining mortality was unpredictable. A similar finding was published more recently by Licker and colleagues [2], who evaluated 654 patients and were able to predict only 22% of observed mortality. This task has become even more complex within the past several years, as attention to patients' postoperative quality of life has been included in the preoperative risk calculus, and the multimodality approach to lung cancer requires the surgeon to consider more operative approaches and interdisciplinary therapies. In this setting, preoperative risk stratification becomes an even more necessary tool in the surgeon's armamentarium to tailor appropriate therapy to individual patients. Other unidentified or unrecognized factors must play a role in these outcomes. Recently identified factors include diffusion capacity for carbon monoxide (DLCO) and cardiopulmonary exercise capacity.

Diffusion capacity

DLCO is a proxy measurement for alveolar oxygen exchange of atmospheric oxygen that capitalizes on carbon monoxide's (CO) strong affinity for hemoglobin. Patients inhale gas containing a known concentration of CO to total lung capacity, hold the breath for 10 seconds, and then completely exhale (forced vital capacity, or FVC).

* Corresponding author.
E-mail address: alexit_2000@yahoo.com (A. Brunelli).

1547-4127/08/$ - see front matter
doi:10.1016/j.thorsurg.2007.11.001

The calculated difference in CO concentration yields the diffusing capacity. DLCO is influenced by the following variables: alveolar membrane area, the pressure of the diffusing gas, and the carrying capacity of the circulating blood volume. The measurement is affected by the patient's age, sex, height, and hemoglobin level [3]. Unlike spirometric measurements, assessment of DLCO is generally not influenced by patient effort.

In the 1950s and 1960s there was initial recognition of diffusing capacity for carbon monoxide as a physiologic marker of respiratory function. Severe emphysema, with an accompanying low DLCO, was shown to be associated with poor long-term survival [4]. Several reports demonstrated that DLCO decreased after lung resection [5–8]. Ultimately Boushy and colleagues [9] showed that a low DLCO anecdotally was associated with an increased incidence of operative mortality after major lung resection.

Using what at the time was a large database of lung resection patients, Ferguson and colleagues [10] first demonstrated DLCO to be an independent predictor of postoperative mortality and pulmonary morbidity. The investigators identified increased mortality in patients with a DLCO of less than 60% of normal, as well as a two- to threefold increased risk of pulmonary morbidity if the DLCO was less than 80%. Rather than using the absolute value for DLCO, which can often be misleading, percentages for DLCO were calculated based upon normal values, which accounted for both the height and age of patients, and were subsequently corrected for serum hemoglobin. Similar findings were subsequently reported by Markos and colleagues [11] and Pierce and colleagues [12].

In parallel to estimations of postoperative predicted spirometric values, there has been increasing interest in using the predicted postoperative (ppo) value for DLCO rather than the actual DLCO as a further refinement for estimating the patient's postoperative pulmonary reserve, especially in patients who have borderline or abnormal preoperative exams. A variety of methods can be used to estimate postoperative lung function, many of which are detailed in "Assessing regional lung function," by Koegelenberg and Bolliger elsewhere in this issue. Currently, a value for ppoDLCO of 40% is used to distinguish between normal risk and higher risk patients [13,14].

One issue that is controversial is whether DLCO should be measured routinely, or only in patients who have compromised spirometric function. Forced expiratory volume in the first second of expiration (FEV_1) and DLCO are thought to be complimentary pulmonary function tests, given that each assesses a distinct physiologic function of the lungs: airflow versus gas-exchange. FEV_1 is still considered by many surgeons to be the definitive pulmonary function test to perform prior to lung resection, and many clinicians will not perform DLCO measurement on patients' whose FEV_1 is greater than 80% of predicted normal. In the Thoracic Database of the Society of Thoracic Surgeons, only 57% of patients undergoing major lung resection from 2000 to 2006 had DLCO values reported (unpublished data). More striking was the finding from the European Thoracic Surgery Database that only 23% of surgeons reported DLCO values for their major lung resection patients [15]. Recent guidelines support this algorithm [16,17]. However, recent data show that DLCO is very important in predicting postoperative complications, even in patients without impaired FEV_1 (less than 80% of predicted) or chronic obstructive lung disease (as defined by an FEV_1/FVC ratio less than 0.7) [14,18]. In fact, DLCO is an equally strong predictor of postoperative complications in patients with and without chronic obstructive pulmonary disease (COPD). These findings indicate that DLCO should be routinely measured during preoperative evaluation, regardless of whether or not the spirometric evaluation is abnormal.

Brunelli and colleagues [19] recently found discrepancies between ppoDLCO and observed postoperative DLCO. Their study suggested that the correlation between predicted and observed values changes over time: ppoDLCO overestimates actual postoperative DLCO in the immediate postoperative period; predicted and actual postoperative DLCO are similar at 1 month after resection; and ppoDLCO underestimates observed postoperative DLCO at 3 months after resection. The investigators cautioned against the use of ppoDLCO as a determinant of intermediate term outcomes. Furthermore, Wang and colleagues [20] demonstrated that preoperative DLCO is not a predictor of long-term mortality after major lung resection. However, Bousamra and colleagues [21] showed that a low preoperative diffusing capacity is related to an increased frequency of readmission to the hospital and a worse long-term quality of life.

Many patients undergoing major lung resection for cancer receive preoperative chemotherapy. Recent reports suggest that chemotherapy can be associated with a 10% to 20% reduction in DLCO, despite stable or improved spirometric values after the therapy [22–24]. The mechanism is presumably related to pneumonitis, although patients did not have demonstrable respiratory symptoms. The decrease in DLCO was associated with an increase in postoperative respiratory complications [23,24]. Assessment of pulmonary status after induction therapy and prior to resection is recommended to ensure that the operative risk has not increased as a result of newly impaired DLCO. If such impairment exists, the benefit of waiting for the DLCO to improve must be weighed against the risk of cancer progression and increased technical surgical difficulty.

Exercise tests

Exercise testing is increasingly used to assess the aerobic reserve of lung resection candidates. These tests have the capability to assess the oxygen transport system in its wholeness and to detect possible deficits that may predispose to postoperative complications. Patients with marginal aerobic reserve have greater difficulty handling the multiple pathophysiologic changes that accompany major surgical procedures [25]. In fact, in the normal postoperative period, a rise in oxygen consumption of a variable extent is expected [26]. The onset of a complication may further increase the oxygen requirements beyond that which the patient can provide, inducing an oxygen debt. If this debt remains critically high over specified periods of time, then a multiorgan failure may ensue [27].

Exercise is attractive before surgery because it increases utilization of oxygen peripherally and requires the entire interlocking lung-heart-vascular oxygen transport system to react [28]. In the lung, exercise determines an increase in ventilation, oxygen consumption per unit time (VO_2), carbon dioxide excretion, and blood flow, similar to those experienced after lung resection. Therefore, the potential exists to evaluate much of the cardiopulmonary system with just one test.

Exercise tests may be grouped in two classes: low-technology and high-technology tests. The first type includes simple, economic tests requiring few resources and personnel; the second type includes more sophisticated and expensive tests that are, however, much more informative about the pathophysiology of the cardiorespiratory system. Both types of exercises may play a role in the preoperative work-up of surgical patients and are not mutually exclusive, but rather may complement each other in a way that is yet mostly unexplored.

Low-technology exercise tests

The most commonly used and studied inexpensive tests are the walking test and the stair-climbing test.

Walking test

Because one's ability to ambulate independently often indicates functional status, assessment of distance ambulated in a specific time period has been reported as a possible method of evaluating performance. The distance walked in 2, 6, and 12 minutes has been studied, with the consensus that the use of a standard time, rather than a standard distance, applies a more uniform test of endurance [29].

Distance walked in 12 minutes was shown to be highly reliable in estimating peak oxygen consumption (VO_2max) in healthy subjects [30], although a lower correlation was observed in patients with COPD [29]. In a more recent study, a strong correlation was found between VO_2max and distance walked in 6 minutes in a population of transplant candidates with end-staged lung disease [31].

In 1984, Bagg [32] described the findings in 30 patients with lung cancer who were exercised with a 12-minute walking test before surgery. No relationship was found between the distance walked and the level of dyspnea experienced by each subject during exercise and the occurrence of postoperative complications. In 1989, Markos and colleagues [11] did not find the distance walked in 12 minutes predictive of cardiopulmonary complications after lung resection.

In a more recent paper from Holden and colleagues [33], the distance walked in 6 minutes was predictive of mortality within 90 days of operation in a group of patients with FEV_1 less than 1.6 L. A distance longer than 1,000 feet was predictive of survival with a sensitivity of 100%, a negative predictive value of 100%, and a positive predictive value of 85%. Pierce and colleagues [12] reported that a 6-minute walking distance was predictive of respiratory failure, but not of other complications or mortality, in a series of candidates for lung resection for lung cancer.

The shuttle walk test has been reported to be more reproducible and more highly correlated with VO_2max estimated by formal exercise testing than the 6-minute walk test [34–37]. It has been estimated by regression analysis that 25 shuttles on the shuttle walk test indicate a VO_2max of 10 mL/kg per minute [34], and therefore this cut-off value has been suggested in the functional algorithm proposed by the British Thoracic Society [38] as a selection criteria for surgery.

However, Win and colleagues recently [39] did not find any statistically significant difference in shuttle walk distance between patients with and without complications after lung resection. They concluded that this test should not be used to predict poor surgical outcome in lung cancer patients, contrary to current recommendations from the British Thoracic Society [38]. More recently, the same investigators found that this test tends to underestimate exercise capacity at the lower range, compared with peak oxygen consumption, and the performance at a shuttle walk test should not be used alone to exclude patients from an operation, without a formal exercise test with VO_2max measurement [40].

Stair climbing test

Stair climbing tests have been used by surgeons for decades [41]. Van Nostrand and colleagues [42] were the first to publish a retrospective series including the stair climb in the preoperative evaluation. They found that patients unable to climb two flights of stairs had a 50% mortality rate after pneumonectomy.

Olsen and colleagues [43] reported a series of 54 patients who performed a stair climb test before lung resection. They found that the ability to climb three flights of stairs most clearly separated those patients with longer hospital stay, postoperative intubation, and greater frequency of complications. Unfortunately, small numbers precluded the possibility to assess the role of stair climbing in predicting fatal cardiopulmonary morbidity.

In a series of high risk patients (FEV_1 less than 1.6 L), Holden and colleagues [33] showed that patients sustaining fatal complications after lung resection climbed fewer steps than those having few or no complications (42 versus 71, $P < .05$). Climbing more than 44 steps was predictive of successful surgical outcome.

In 2001, Girish and colleagues [44] prospectively evaluated 83 patients undergoing thoracotomy or upper abdominal laparotomy surgery, and found that patients with complications climbed significantly fewer flights of stairs than those without complications (2.1 versus 4.4, $P = .00002$). The inability to climb two flights of stairs was associated with a positive predictive value of 80%; conversely, the ability to climb more than five flights of stairs was associated with a negative predictive value of 95%.

Brunelli and colleagues [45] reported the largest series so far, evaluating the role of stair climb in predicting postoperative complications after lung resection. In this prospective study, including 160 lung resection candidates, the investigators standardized the results of the test by expressing the number of steps climbed as altitude in meters, as suggested by Pate and colleagues [46]. The altitude reached when testing stair climbing resulted in the only independent predictor of cardiopulmonary complications after controlling the effect of other variables by logistic regression analysis. In particular, only 6.5% of subjects climbing more than 14 meters in altitude had complications. However, 29% of subjects who climbed between 12 and 14 meters, and 50% of those climbing less than 12 meters, had complications. This progressive increase of cardiopulmonary morbidity rate with the reduction of the altitude climbed preoperatively, indirectly demonstrates that stair climbing is a stressful test capable of revealing severe deficits in maximum aerobic capacity. In the same article, Brunelli and colleagues [45] proved that stair climbing was superior with respect to spirometric variables in discriminating between complicated and noncomplicated patients. In a high-risk group of 17 patients with $ppoFEV_1$ less than 35% or ppoDLCO less than 35%, and who were judged to be operable on the basis of their satisfactory performance at the stair climbing test, the investigators observed only four complications and no mortality. The investigators concluded that this type of exercise should be added as a routine screening test to all lung resection candidates.

The same group from Ancona [47] confirmed the predictive role of stair climbing in a cohort of 109 patients, older than 70 years of age, undergoing pulmonary lobectomy. Patients with complications climbed on average 3 meters less than those without complications ($P = .0004$). The altitude reached at stair climbing test remained an independent significant predictor of complications after logistic regression analysis.

The appeal of symptom-limited stair climbing test resides in its simplicity and brevity (1–2 minutes), the familiarity of the patient with the exercise, and the need of few personnel, expertise, and equipment. Moreover, it has been reported that this test yields higher value of peak VO_2 than cycle-ergometry [33,35,48]. This finding may be explained by the fact that stair climbing is a more stressful exercise than cycling or treadmill, involving a larger muscle mass, and is extremely motivating for the patients who are pushed to reach a visible objective represented by the next landing.

However, although this test is quite effective in predicting complications by uncovering deficits in the cardiopulmonary system, it provides very little information on the causes that are behind the reduced aerobic capacity. For this reason, the authors believe that in order to optimize the preoperative functional evaluation pathways of the lung resection candidates, this test could be ideally used as an initial preoperative screening exercise test in all patients. Nevertheless, in those patients with a poor performance at the stair climbing test (ie, less than 12 meters in altitude), a formal cardiopulmonary exercise test with measurement of peak oxygen consumption should be recommended to define the pathophysiologic basis of their performance and optimize perioperative management.

Exercise oxygen desaturation

Although exercise oximetry has been proposed as a useful tool in the preoperative functional evaluation of the lung resection candidates [16,38], the role of exercise oxygen desaturation (EOD) in risk-stratification has not been defined, and nonunivocal conclusions have been published regarding its definition and its association with early outcome after lung resection [49–51].

In 1995, Rao and colleagues [49] analyzed 299 patients undergoing lung resection, with the aim to compare predictive ability of exercise oximetry (desaturation below 90% while walking on the level and climbing two flights of stairs) and spirometry. The investigators found that EOD was a better discriminant of postoperative respiratory failure, need for intensive care unit admission, prolonged hospital stay, and home oxygen requirement, with respect to traditional spirometry parameters. These findings were confirmed by Ninan and colleagues [50], who studied 46 pneumonectomy patients assessed by exercise oximetry on a stair-stepper apparatus. They found that an EOD below 90% or greater than 4% was associated with longer intensive care unit stay and higher incidence of major complications.

At variance with these results, Varela and colleagues [51] found that oxygen desaturation below 90% during standardized incremental cycle-ergometry was not a significant predictor of postoperative cardiopulmonary morbidity.

In a recent study, Brunelli and colleagues [52] investigated the best cut-off definition of EOD and its role in predicting cardiopulmonary morbidity in 536 patients submitted to major lung resection. They found that a desaturation greater than 4% was significantly associated with postoperative complications, even after adjusting its effect for other factors with regression analysis. On the other hand, an exercise oxygen level below 90% was not a significant discriminant between complicated and noncomplicated patients. Patients experiencing EOD greater than 4% had morbidity and mortality rates of 36% and 8%, respectively (versus 22% and 3%, respectively). The investigators also found that patients with an associated cardiac comorbidity who experienced EOD had a morbidity rate of 51%, and those climbing less than 12 meters with concomitant EOD had a complication rate of 71% and a mortality rate of 29%. The investigators concluded that oxygen desaturation should be regarded as a reliable marker of deficits in the oxygen transport system. For this reason, those patients in whom EOD is observed should be further assessed with a formal cardiopulmonary exercise test (CPET) for a more precise evaluation of their cardiopulmonary system, in order to optimize their perioperative management.

High-technology exercise tests

High-technology exercise testing is another expression for the more commonly used term, cardiopulmonary exercise testing. In CPET, maximal or symptom-limited exercise is performed, usually on a bicycle or treadmill. There are several advantages of CPET over the much simpler "low tech" exercise tests. These tests are performed in a controlled environment with continuous monitoring of various parameters. This ensures easy standardization and good reproducibility of results. Although CPET is more time-consuming than simple stair climbing, 6-minute walk, or shuttle tests, test duration rarely exceed 20 minutes, including recovery time. CPET further offers the safest approach of all exercise modalities, as the patient exercises "on the same spot" and resuscitation equipment can be kept stationary near by. Maximal oxygen consumption is the single most important parameter as a direct measure of work load or exercise capacity. Other important directly measured parameters include: breath rate, tidal volume, carbon dioxide production (VCO_2), pulse rate, blood pressure, and the electrocardiogram. All these parameters, as well as a number of derived parameters such as ventilation and oxygen pulse, are continuously analyzed as they change in response to incremental workloads. This does not only allow assessment of over-all cardiopulmonary reserves, but in case of a limitation of exercise capacity (ie, a reduced VO_2max), to find the reason for this, such as pulmonary, cardiovascular, or musculo-skeletal limitations. If a particular organ system can be incriminated as the limiting factor, specific treatment options can be of benefit, such as optimization of COPD treatment or management of ischemic heart disease.

The importance of VO_2max was suggested by an early small study of 19 subjects, published in 1982 by Eugene and colleagues [53], who found that a VO_2max of less than 1,000 ml was associated with a 75% mortality, whereas as FEV_1 and FVC had no predictive value for postoperative complications. Subsequently, a good number of larger studies by various investigators have confirmed the predictive value of VO_2max measurements, and various cut-off values of VO_2max expressed either in ml/kg per minute or in percent of predicted values have been suggested, which indicate whether patients can safely undergo pulmonary resections, and most importantly, estimate the extent of resection possible [17,46,54–62]. Without discussing these studies in detail, it can be said that there is currently wide consensus that the following cut-off values can be recommended. Expressed in absolute values, a VO_2max of greater than 20 ml/kg per minute qualifies for pneumonectomy, greater than 15 ml/kg per minute for lobectomy, and less than 10 ml/kg per minute indicates high risk for any resection. Expressed in percent of predicted, the respective values are greater than 75%, greater than 60%, and greater than 40%. In addition, Bolliger first suggested the use of predicted postoperative values for VO_2max—well established for FEV_1 and DLCO (see "Assessing regional lung function" by Koegelenberg and Bolliger in this issue)—and found that a calculated value of VO_2max-ppo less than 10 ml/kg per minute was the only parameter which retrospectively identified all three patients who died, in a subgroup of 25 patients at increased risk for postresectional complications [58]. The value of VO_2max-ppo for the prediction of postresectional complications has since been confirmed in a study by Brunelli and colleagues [45].

Algorithm for the assessment of cardio-pulmonary reserves

Although VO_2max is the single most potent parameter to assess cardiopulmonary reserves, it is not recommended as the sole parameter overruling all others. On the one hand, the vast majority of lung resection candidates qualify for safe resections up to a pneumonectomy, measuring simple spirometry and the diffusing capacity, taking their respective ppo-values into consideration, combined with low-technology exercise tests as discussed above. On the other hand, CPET, with its high technology equipment is expensive and therefore not universally available. It is thus highly desirable to have an algorithm according to which patients undergo successive steps, passing from simple to more complex investigations of functional assessment. The most widely used such algorithm initially proposed [63] and subsequently prospectively validated [61] by Bolliger and colleagues is based on cardiac parameters, two pulmonary parameters (FEV_1, DLCO), and VO_2max (Fig. 1). A slightly different algorithm—an unvalidated consensus product—has been proposed in the recent 2nd edition of the American College of Chest Physicians evidence-based practice guidelines for the diagnosis and management of lung cancer [16]. Adherence to such algorithms helps to include rather than to exclude patients from surgery, because patients who are unable to qualify by one single parameter can compensate by having larger reserves in other parameters: that is, a relatively weak FEV_1 can be compensated by a good DLCO [12], VO_2max, or stair climbing ability. Patients who are considered at high risk for any resections will either be deemed inoperable or a decision on an individual basis will have to be made as to the risk both patient and doctor are prepared to take. Thanks to the advances in surgical techniques (minimally invasive procedures, combination of lung cancer surgery with lung volume reduction surgery [64], and the ongoing improvement in postoperative care), the limits of functional operability are constantly being lowered, thus allowing resections in patients who would have been deemed inoperable a few years ago.

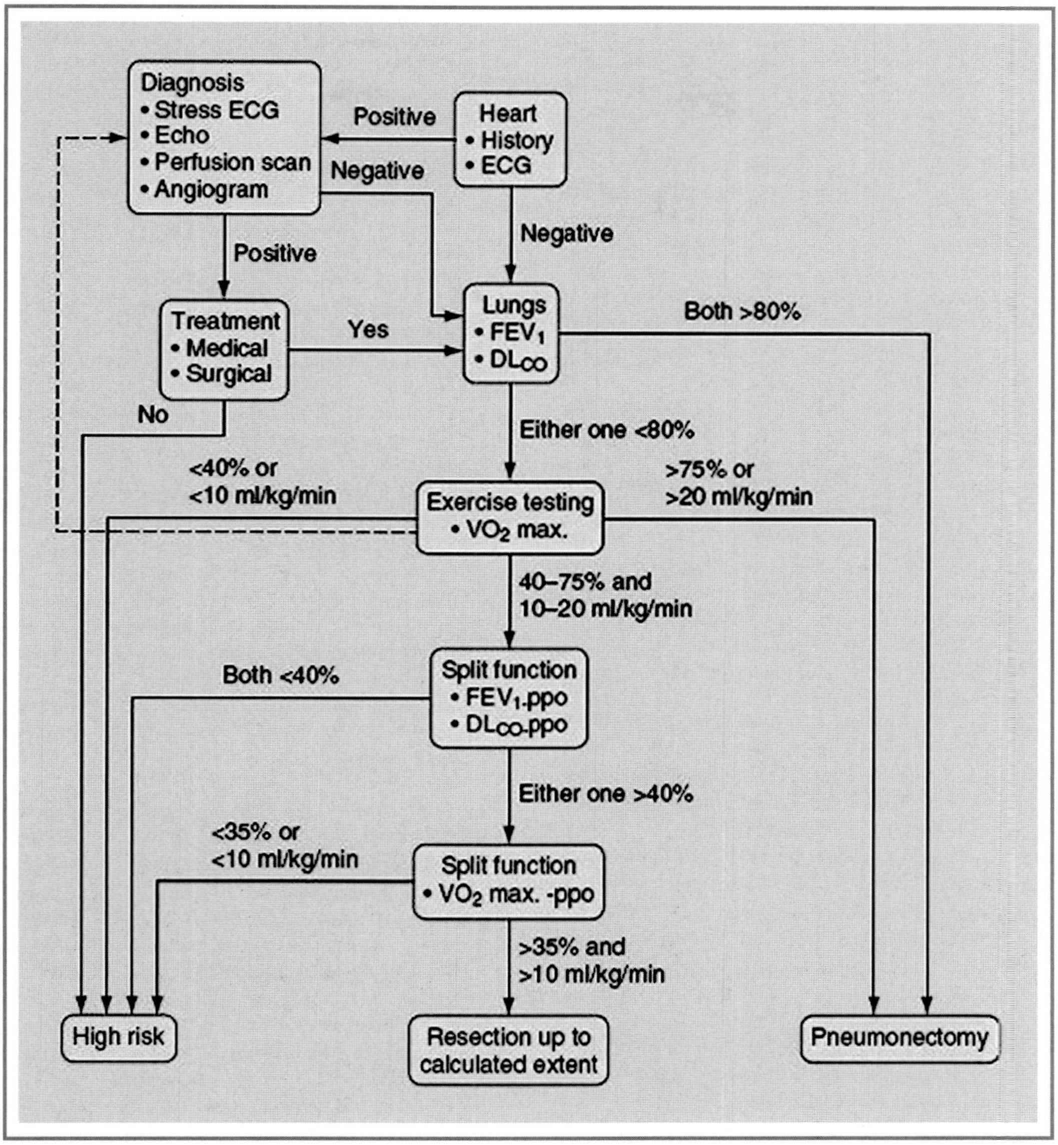

Fig. 1. Algorithm for the assessment of cardiorespiratory reserve and operability of candidates for lung resection. Patients undergo successive steps, from top to bottom, until they either qualify for varying extents of resection or are deemed high risk. A safety loop for patients with possible cardiac disease detected on exercise testing (signs or symptoms of myocardial ischemia) is shown by the dashed line in the upper left-hand corner. Split lung function testing allows a more accurate estimate of predicted postoperative function (see article by Koegelenberg and Bolliger on assessing regional lung function elsewhere in this issue). This is usually calculated by means of anatomic calculations, CT scan, or the use of split perfusion scanning. Note that all percentages refer to percentages predicted. Care must be taken to understand that ppo calculations by implication take the calculated extent of resection into account, and that this may vary from a wedge resection to a lobectomy up to a pneumonectomy. (*Adapted from* Schuurmans MM, Diacon AH, Bolliger CT. Functional evaluation before lung resection. Clin Chest Med 2002;23:159–72; with permission).

References

[1] Kohman LJ, Meyer JA, Ikins PM, et al. Random versus predictable risks of mortality after thoracotomy for lung cancer. J Thorac Cardiovasc Surg 1986;91:551–4.

[2] Licker M, de Perrot M, Höhn L, et al. Perioperative mortality and major cardio-pulmonary complications after lung surgery for non-small cell carcinoma. Eur J Cardiothorac Surg 1999;15:314–9.

[3] Levitzky M. Pulmonary physiology. 5th edition. McGraw-Hill; USA 1999. Chapters 1, 3, 6, 7.

[4] Bates DV, Knott JM, Christie RV. Respiratory function in emphysema in relation to prognosis. Q J Med 1956;25:137–57.

[5] Bates DV, McIlroy MB. Respiratory function after pneumonectomy. Thorax 1956;11:303–11.

[6] Curtis JK, Bauer H, Loomans S, et al. Pulmonary diffusion capacity studies. II. Clinical results using a modified carbon monoxide breathholding technique. Am J Med Sci 1958;236:57–64.

[7] Burrows B, Harrison RW, Adams WE, et al. The postpneumonectomy state: clinical and physiologic observations in thirty-six cases. Am J Med 1960;28:281–97.

[8] Dietiker F, Lester W, Burrows B. The effects of thoracic surgery on the pulmonary diffusing capacity. Am Rev Respir Dis 1960;81:830–8.

[9] Boushy SF, Helgason AH, Billig DM, et al. Clinical, physiologic, and morphologic examination of the lung in patients with bronchogenic carcinoma and the relation of the findings to postoperative deaths. Am Rev Respir Dis 1970;101:685–95.

[10] Ferguson MK, Little L, Rizzo L, et al. Diffusing capacity predicts morbidity and mortality after pulmonary resection. J Thorac Cardiovasc Surg 1988;96:894–900.

[11] Markos J, Mullan BP, Hillman DR, et al. Preoperative assessment as a predictor of mortality and morbidity after lung resection. Am Rev Respir Dis 1989; 139:902–10.

[12] Pierce RJ, Copland JM, Sharpe K, et al. Preoperative risk evaluation for lung cancer resection: predicted postoperative product as a predictor of surgical mortality. Am J Respir Crit Care Med 1994;150:947–55.

[13] Ferguson MK, Reeder LB, Mick R. Optimizing selection of patients for major lung resection. J Thorac Cardiovasc Surg 1995;109:275–83.

[14] Brunelli A, Refai M, Salati M, et al. Carbon monoxide lung diffusion capacity improves risk stratification in patients without airflow limitation: evidence for systematic measurement before lung resection. Eur J Cardiothorac Surg 2006;29:567–70.

[15] Berrisford R, Brunelli A, Rocco G, et al. Audit and guidelines committee of the European Society of Thoracic Surgeons; European Association of Cardiothoracic Surgeons. The European Thoracic Surgery Database project: modeling the risk of in-hospital death following lung resection. Eur J Cardiothorac Surg 2005;28:306–11.

[16] Colice GL, Shafazand S, Griffin JP, et al. Physiologic evaluation of the patient with lung cancer being considered for resectional surgery. ACCP Evidenced-based clinical practice guidelines (2nd edition). Chest 2007;132:161S–77S.

[17] Loewen GM, Watson D, Kohman L, et al, Cancer and Leukemia Group B. Preoperative exercise VO2 measurement for lung resection candidates: results of Cancer and Leukemia Group B Protocol 9238. J Thorac Oncol 2007;2:619–25.

[18] Ferguson MK, Vigneswaran WT. Diffusing capacity predicts morbidity after lung resection in patients without obstructive lung disease. Ann Thorac Surg, in press.

[19] Brunelli A, Refai M, Salati M, et al. Predicted versus observed FEV1 and DLCO after major lung resection: a prospective evaluation at different postoperative periods. Ann Thorac Surg 2007;83:1134–9.

[20] Wang J, Olak J, Ferguson MK. Diffusing capacity predicts operative mortality but not long-term survival after resection for lung cancer. J Thorac Cardiovasc Surg 1999;117:581–7.

[21] Bousamra M 2nd, Presberg KW, Chammas JH, et al. Early and late morbidity in patients undergoing pulmonary resection with low diffusion capacity. Ann Thorac Surg 1996;62:968–75.

[22] Dimopoulou I, Galani H, Dafni U, et al. A prospective study of pulmonary function in patients treated with paclitaxel and carboplatin. Cancer 2002;94: 452–8.

[23] Leo F, Solli P, Spaggiari L, et al. Respiratory function changes after chemotherapy: an additional risk for postoperative respiratory complications? Ann Thorac Surg 2004;77:260–5.

[24] Takeda S, Funakoshi Y, Kadota Y, et al. Fall in diffusing capacity associated with induction therapy for lung cancer: a predictor of postoperative complication? Ann Thorac Surg 2006;82:232–6.

[25] Gump FE, Martin P, Kinney JM. Oxygen consumption and caloric expenditure in surgical patients. Surg Gynecol Obstet 1973;137:499–513.

[26] Gilbreth EM, Weisman IM. Role of exercise stress testing in preoperative evaluation of patients for lung resection. Clin Chest Med 1994;15:389–403.

[27] Shoemaker WC, Appel PL, Kram HB. Tissue oxygen debt as a determinant of lethal and non-lethal postoperative organ failure. Crit Care Med 1988; 16:1117–20.

[28] Olsen GN. The evolving role of exercise testing prior to lung resection. Chest 1989;95:218–25.

[29] McGavin CF, Gupta SP, McHardy GJR. Twelve minute walking test for assessing disability in chronic bronchitis. BMJ 1997;1:822–3.

[30] Cooper KH. A means of assessing maximal oxygen intake. JAMA 1968;203:135–8.

[31] Cahalin L, Pappagianopoulos P, Prevost S, et al. The relationship of 6-min walk test to maximal oxygen consumption in transplant candidates with end-stage lung disease. Chest 1995;108:452–9.

[32] Bagg LR. The 12-min walking distance: its use in the preoperative assessment of patients with bronchial carcinoma before lung resection. Respiration 1984; 46:342–5.

[33] Holden DA, Rice TW, Stelmach K, et al. Exercise testing, 6-min walk, and stair climb in the evaluation of patients at high risk for pulmonary resection. Chest 1992;102:1774–9.

[34] Singh SJ, Morgan MD, Hardman AE, et al. Comparison of oxygen uptake during a conventional treadmill test and the shuttle walking test in chronic airflow limitation. Eur Respir J 1994;7:2016–20.

[35] Swinburn CR, Wakefield JM, Jones PW. Performance, ventilation and oxygen consumption in three different types of exercise test in patients with chronic obstructive lung disease. Thorax 1985;40:581–6.

[36] Morgan AD. Simple exercise testing. Respir Med 1989;83:383–7.

[37] Bernstein ML, Despars JA, Singh NP, et al. Reanalysis of the 12-minute walk in patients with chronic obstructive lung disease. Chest 1994;105:163–7.

[38] British Thoracic Society, Society of Cardiothoracic Surgeons of Great Britain and Ireland Working Party. BTS guidelines: guidelines on the selection of patients with lung cancer for surgery. Thorax 2001;56:89–108.

[39] Win T, Jackson A, Groves AM, et al. Relationship between shuttle walk test and lung cancer surgical outcome. Eur J Cardiothorac Surg 2004;26:1216–9.

[40] Win T, Jackson A, Groves AM, et al. Comparison of shuttle walk and measured peak oxygen consumption in patients with operable lung cancer. Thorax 2006;61:57–60.

[41] Sonders CR. The clinical evaluation of the patient for thoracic surgery. Surg Clin North Am 1961;41: 545–58.

[42] Van Nostrand D, Kjelsberg MO, Humphrey EW. Preresectional evaluation of risk from pneumonectomy. Surg Gynecol Obstet 1968;127:306–12.

[43] Olsen GN, Bolton JWR, Weiman DS, et al. Stair climbing as an exercise test to predict the postoperative complications of lung resection. Chest 1991;99: 587–90.

[44] Girish M, Trayner E, Damman O, et al. Symptom-limited stair climbing as a predictor of postoperative cardiopulmonary complications after high-risk surgery. Chest 2001;120:1147–51.

[45] Brunelli A, Refai M, Monteverde M, et al. Stair climbing test predicts cardiopulmonary complications after lung resection. Chest 2002;121:1106–10.

[46] Pate P, Tenholder MF, Griffin JP, et al. Preoperative assessment of the high-risk patient for lung resection. Ann Thorac Surg 1996;61:1494–500.

[47] Brunelli A, Monteverde M, Refai M, et al. Stair climbing test as a predictor of cardiopulmonary complications after pulmonary lobectomy in the elderly. Ann Thorac Surg 2004;77:266–70.

[48] Pollock M, Roa J, Benditt J, et al. Estimation of ventilatory reserve by stair climbing: a study in patients with chronic airflow obstruction. Chest 1993;104: 1378–83.

[49] Rao V, Todd TRJ, Kuus A, et al. Exercise oximetry versus spirometry in the assessment of risk prior to lung resection. Ann Thorac Surg 1995;60:603–9.

[50] Ninan M, Sommers KE, Landreneau RJ, et al. Standardized exercise oximetry predicts postpneumonectomy outcome. Ann Thorac Surg 1997;64:328–32.

[51] Varela G, Cordovilla R, Jimenez MF, et al. Utility of standardized exercise oximetry to predict cardiopulmonary morbidity after lung resection. Eur J Cardiothorac Surg 2001;19:351–4.

[52] Brunelli A, Refai M, Xiumé F, et al. Oxygen desaturation during maximal stair climbing test and postoperative complications. Eur J Cardiothorac Surg, in press.

[53] Eugene J, Brown SE, Light RW, et al. Maximum oxygen consumption: a physiological guide to pulmonary resection. Surg Forum 1982;33:260–2.

[54] Smith TP, Kinasewitz GT, Tucker WY, et al. Exercise capacity as a predictor of post-thoracotomy morbidity. Am Rev Respir Dis 1984;129:730–4.

[55] Bechard D, Wetstein L. Assessment of exercise oxygen consumption as preoperative criterion for lung resection. Ann Thorac Surg 1987;44:344–9.

[56] Morice RC, Peters EJ, Ryan MB, et al. Exercise testing in the evaluation of patients at high risk for complications from lung resection. Chest 1992;101:356–61.

[57] Walsh GL, Morice RC, Putnam JB Jr, et al. Resection of lung cancer is justified in high risk patients selected by exercise oxygen consumption. Ann Thorac Surg 1994;58:704–10.

[58] Bolliger CT, Wyser C, Roser H, et al. Lung scanning and exercise testing for the prediction of postoperative performance in lung resection candidates at increased risk for complications. Chest 1995;108: 341–8.

[59] Bolliger CT, Jordan P, Soler M, et al. Exercise capacity as a predictor of postoperative complications in lung resection candidates. Am J Respir Crit Care Med 1995;151(5):1472–80.

[60] Wyser C, Stulz P, Soler M, et al. Prospective evaluation of an algorithm for the functional assessment of lung resection candidates. Am J Respir Crit Care Med 1999;159:1450–6.

[61] Brutsche M, Spiliopoulos A, Bolliger CT, et al. Exercise capacity and extent of resection as predictors of surgical risk in lung cancer. Eur Respir J 2000; 15:828–32.

[62] Win T, Jackson A, Sharples L, et al. Cardiopulmonary exercise tests and lung cancer surgical outcome. Chest 2005;127:1159–65.

[63] Bolliger CT, Perruchoud AP. Functional evaluation of the lung resection candidate. Eur Respir J 1998; 11:198–212.

[64] Choong CK, Meyers BF, Battafarano RJ. Lung cancer resection combined with lung volume reduction in patients with severe emphysema. J Thorac Cardiovasc Surg 2004;127:1323–31.

ELSEVIER
SAUNDERS

Thorac Surg Clin 18 (2008) 19–29

THORACIC
SURGERY
CLINICS

Assessing Regional Lung Function

Coenraad F.N. Koegelenberg, MBChB, FCP(SA), MRCP(UK)*,
Chris T. Bolliger, MD, PhD

Division of Pulmonology, Department of Medicine, Faculty of Health Sciences, University of Stellenbosch, Francie van Zijl Drive, Health Sciences Complex, Tygerberg 7505, Cape Town, South Africa

The assessment of regional lung function forms an integral part of the preoperative evaluation of pulmonary resection candidates who have impaired lung function. The mortality and morbidity related to pulmonary resection are dependent not only on the extent of resection, comorbid diseases, and cardiopulmonary reserves, but also on the post-resectional lung function [1,2]. Clinicians involved in the preoperative evaluation of these patients need to comprehend and utilize the various means of estimating the relative contribution of the pulmonary parenchyma earmarked for resection. In this article the authors introduce the concept of predicted postoperative (PPO) lung function, review the different techniques available for estimating regional or relative lung function, and conclude with a practical approach to the assessment of regional lung function and the prediction of postoperative pulmonary reserves prior to pulmonary resection.

Predicted postoperative lung function

Patients who have impaired pulmonary functions—defined as a forced expiratory volume in 1 second (FEV_1) or a carbon monoxide diffusing capacity (DL_{CO}) of less than 80% of predicted—warrant more extensive evaluation of their pulmonary reserves [1–4]. Further investigations should ideally include integrative cardiopulmonary exercise testing [4], and are best guided by a validated algorithm (Fig. 1 is one example of such an algorithm). A decision regarding operability is then based not only on the preoperative percentage of predicted for spirometric values (most importantly FEV_1), the diffusion capacity of the lung (DL_{CO}), or the patient's exercise capacity (maximum or peak oxygen uptake [$\dot{V}O_2$ max]), but more importantly on the PPO values of these parameters. The calculations rely on the ability to estimate the contribution of the parenchyma to be resected relative to the total lung function. The PPO value (see Fig. 1) for any particular parameter, be it a spirometric volume, diffusion capacity, or oxygen uptake, is equal to the preoperative values × (1 − fractional contribution of tissue earmarked for resection) [1–4]. There are essentially four validated ways of estimating the relative functional contribution or split function (and thus to calculate the PPO values): anatomic calculation, split radionucleotide perfusion scanning, quantitative CT scanning, and dynamic perfusion MRI.

Anatomical calculations

Historical perspective

Anatomic calculations of the PPO values are by far the simplest and oldest techniques of predicting regional lung function. Jacobaeus and colleagues [5] were the first to attempt separate functional analysis of the right and left lung when they introduced bronchospirometry in 1932. This technique was used more extensively after the development by Carlens [6] in 1949 of the double-lumen catheter, which allowed separate analysis of the ventilation of the left and right lung. Numerous refinements of this technique were described up to 1970, after which it was largely abandoned in favor of scintigraphic

* Corresponding author.
E-mail address: coeniefn@sun.ac.za (C.F.N. Koegelenberg).

1547-4127/08/$ - see front matter
doi:10.1016/j.thorsurg.2007.10.001

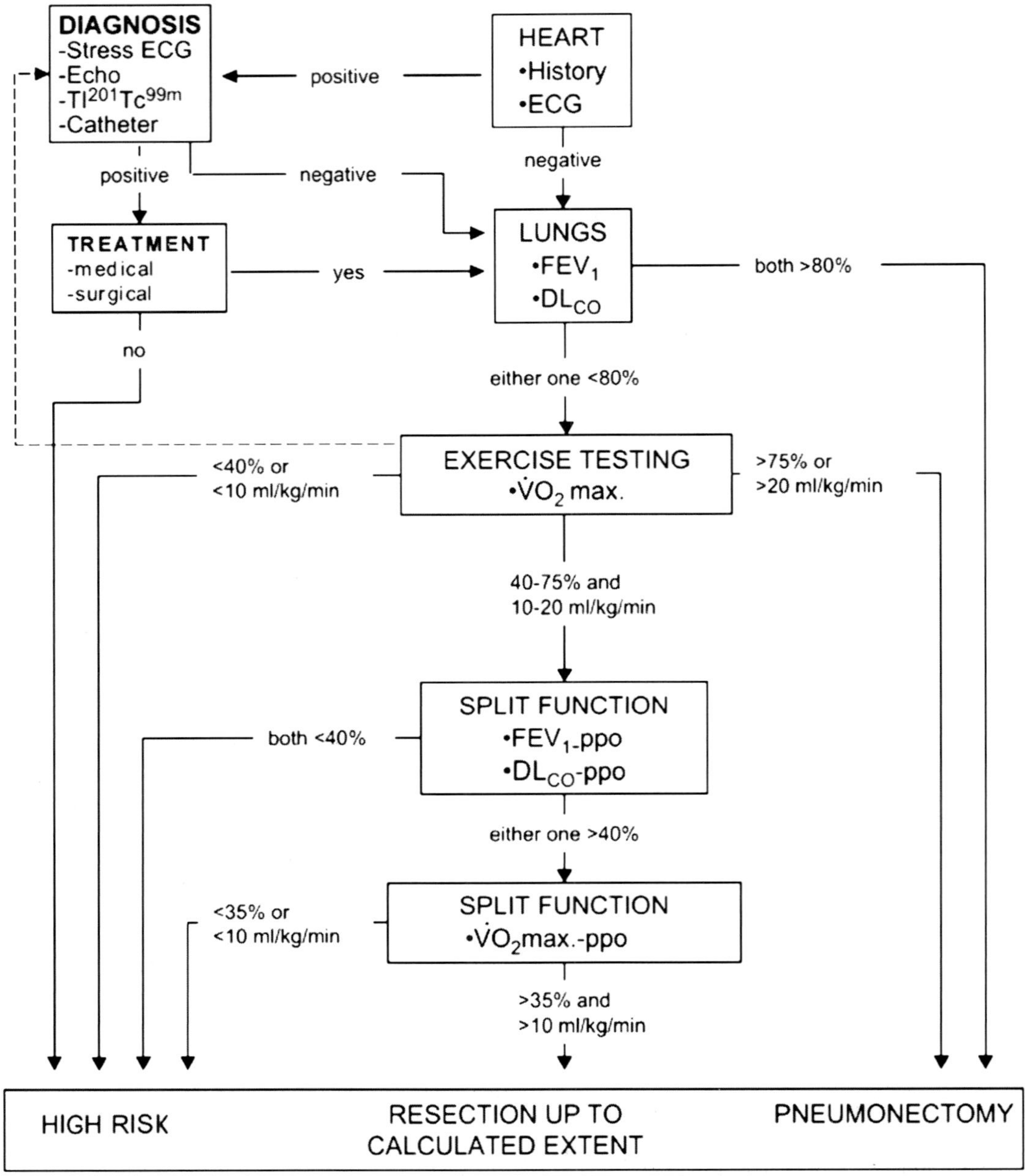

Fig. 1. Algorithm for the assessment of cardiorespiratory reserve and operability of lung resection candidates. Patients undergo successive steps from top to bottom until they either qualify for varying extents of resection or are deemed high risk. A safety loop for patients with possible cardiac disease detected on exercise testing (signs or symptoms of myocardial ischemia) is shown by the dashed line in the upper left hand corner. Split lung function testing allows a more accurate estimate of predicted postoperative (PPO) function. This is usually calculated by means of anatomical calculations, split radionucleotide perfusion scanning, quantitative CT scan, or dynamic perfusion MRI. Note that all cut-off values that are expressed as percentages in this figure refer to percentages of preoperative predicted values. Care must be taken to understand that PPO calculations by implication take the calculated extent of resection into account, and that this may vary from a wedge resection to a lobectomy right up to a pneumonectomy. $\dot{V}O_2$ max, maximal oxygen consumption. PPO values = Preoperative values × (1-fractional contribution of parenchyma earmarked for resection). (*Adapted from* Bolliger CT, Perruchoud AP. Functional evaluation of the lung resection candidate. Eur Respir J 1998;11:206; with permission.)

techniques [3]. Anatomical calculations were, however, revived in the mid 1990s, and subsequently firmly re-established as reasonable predictors of postresectional pulmonary function [7–9].

Modern application

Anatomical calculations can be based either on the number of segments to be removed, thereby estimating PPO function as the fraction of the segments remaining [7,8], or similarly on the number of subsegments [10]. Further distinctions between occluded and patent segments or subsegments are often made, whereby the loss of occluded segments is disregarded [9,10]. Formulae based on these principles and tested in prospective studies, include the following [7–10]:

- Number of segments (S): PPO function = preoperative function x (1 − y/19), where y is the number of segments to be removed, and 19 the total number of segments
- Number of functional segments (FS): PPO function = preoperative function (1 − y/z), where y is the number of functional segments to be removed, and z the total number of functional segments
- Number of subsegments (SS): PPO function = preoperative function x [1 – (b – n)/(42 – n)], where n is the number of obstructed and b the total number of subsegments in the resected lobe; it is assumed that b = 6, 4, 12 in the right upper, middle and lower lobes, respectively, and 10 each in the left upper and lower lobes

In clinical practice, the PPO FEV_1 is most frequently estimated by means of the segmental formula. For a right upper lobectomy, for example, PPO FEV_1 would be equal to the preoperative $FEV_1 \times (16/19)$, provided that the segments are all endoscopically patent. If a patient who has an actual preoperative FEV_1 of 2.20 l (59.5% of a predicted 3.70 l) undergoes this procedure, then the PPO FEV_1 will be $2.20 \times 16/19 = 1.85$ l (50.0% of a predicted 3.70 l). The PPO DL_{CO} and $\dot{V}O_2$ max are calculated in a similar fashion.

Correlation of predicted postoperative function based on anatomical calculations with actual postoperative lung function

Studies comparing PPO estimations based on the various anatomical calculations (S, FS, and SS) with actual postoperative lung function are limited. Bolliger and colleagues [9] found remarkably similar (and equally significant) correlations when they studied these calculations in 44 pulmonary resection candidates. They were able to show a correlation coefficient (r) of 0.88 when comparing estimations to measured lung functions 6 months postoperatively for FEV_1, 0.85 to 0.86 for forced expiratory vital capacity (FVC), 0.84 to 0.85 for DL_{CO}, and 0.75 for $\dot{V}O_2$ max (Table 1). Subanalyses of the study data showed that anatomical calculations were much less accurate at predicting PPO function following pneumonectomy ($r = 0.47$–0.59 for FEV_1) than lobectomy ($r = 0.87$–0.89 for FEV_1), as depicted in Table 2. Stratifying patients according to the presence or absence of obstructive airflow limitation (FEV_1/FVC <0.7) did not alter the correlations.

Radionucleotide perfusion scanning

Background

Radiospirometry for the regional analysis of ventilation was first described in the 1950s, and preceded the use of perfusion scanning [11]. In 1972, Kristersson and colleagues [12] used xenon-133 to accurately predict the functional loss after pneumonectomy and lobectomy. Numerous subsequent studies validated the use of this modality, and the functional loss as predicted by radiospirometry was considered accurate as long as the resection involved more than three segments. In a landmark study by Olsen and colleagues [13] split perfusion scans using intravenous technetium-99 macroaggregates were shown to accurately predict functional loss (FEV_1) 3 months postpneumonectomy. Many authors subsequently confirmed the feasibility of estimating ventilatory function by perfusion scanning. Radionucleotide perfusion scanning eventually replaced radiospirometry as the investigation of choice, given its general availability, ease of performance, and greater reproducibility [14].

Technical aspects

Most institutions use intravenous technetium-99m macroaggregated albumin as the radiopharmaceutical of choice with regards to pulmonary perfusion. These particles are trapped in the pulmonary capillary bed, and emit gamma rays proportional to regional perfusion. In order to obtain the maximum information regarding regional lung perfusion, patients should be scanned in the sitting position and in four projections (anterior, posterior, left posterior oblique, and

Table 1
Data from a prospective study of 44 pulmonary resection candidates. The comparison of five different methods to estimate PPO function for the parameters FEV_1, FVC, DL_{CO}, and $\dot{V}O_2$ max are shown

		A	B	Diff. A-B	p	r	Limits of agreement
FEV_1	CT	1.79	1.92	−0.13	0.001	0.91	−0.65–0.37
	Q	1.88	1.92	−0.04	0.330	0.92	−0.50–0.43
	S	1.71	1.92	−0.21	0.000	0.88	−0.79–0.38
	FS	1.78	1.92	−0.14	0.004	0.88	−0.71–0.44
	SS	1.79	1.92	−0.13	0.007	0.88	−0.71–0.46
FVC	CT	2.64	2.84	−0.20	0.003	0.86	−1.19–0.72
	Q	2.77	2.84	−0.07	0.239	0.90	−0.85–0.71
	S	2.54	2.84	−0.30	0.000	0.86	−1.25–0.63
	FS	2.65	2.84	−0.19	0.010	0.85	−1.16–0.77
	SS	2.65	2.84	−0.19	0.011	0.86	−1.12–0.75
DL_{CO}, ml/min/mmHg	CT	19.93	21.68	−1.75	0.002	0.84	−8.72–5.08
	Q	20.98	21.68	−0.70	0.389	0.85	−7.21–6.31
	S	19.17	21.68	−2.51	0.000	0.84	−9.36–4.73
	FS	20.04	21.68	−1.64	0.010	0.84	−8.32–5.48
	SS	20.14	21.68	−1.54	0.018	0.85	−8.32–5.68
$\dot{V}O_2$ max, ml/kg/min	CT	14.32	16.51	−2.19	0.000	0.77	−7.70–3.02
	Q	15.01	16.51	−1.50	0.000	0.85	−5.85–2.85
	S	13.59	16.51	−2.92	0.000	0.75	−8.52–2.66
	FS	14.26	16.51	−2.25	0.000	0.75	−7.77–3.26
	SS	14.28	16.51	−2.23	0.000	0.75	−7.81–3.35

Abbreviations: A, PPO value; B, measured value 6 months postoperatively; p value, paired t test between A and B; r, correlation coefficient between A and B, limits of agreement: two standard deviations from mean difference between A and B; Q, pulmonary perfusion scanning.

Adapted from Bolliger CT, Guckel C, Engel H, et al. Prediction of functional reserves after lung resection: comparison between quantitative CT, scintigraphy, and anatomy. Respiration 2002;69(6):485; with permission.

right posterior oblique). Scans should be acquired with 5×10^5 counts per image each on a one-head gamma camera (known as a Single Photon Emission CT or SPECT scan) [4,9]. Quantification is performed by means of a system-integrated region-ratio program in the anterior and posterior projections for right-left lung quantification (geometric mean), in the left posterior oblique projection for left lung lobar quantification and the right posterior oblique projection for right lung lobar quantification [9]. An example of such a regional perfusion scan is given in Fig. 2.

Correlation of predicted postoperative function based on radionucleotide perfusion scanning with actual postoperative lung function

Radionucleotide perfusion scanning remains the gold standard for predicting postoperative lung function, although recent studies have certainly challenged this assumption [15–18]. In a prospective study by Bolliger and coworkers [9], radionucleotide perfusion scanning outperformed calculations based on quantitative CT scanning and anatomy with regards to the range of functional parameters (see Tables 1 and 2). Estimates of PPO function based on perfusion scans consistently exhibited the highest correlations with postoperatively measured values for FEV_1 ($r = 0.92$), FVC ($r = 0.90$), DL_{CO} ($r = 0.85$), and $\dot{V}O_2$ max ($r = 0.85$). For $\dot{V}O_2$ max, the radionuclide-based predictions were lower than the measured values, but still closer to the measured values than CT-derived or anatomical calculations. Subanalyses of the Bolliger group's data showed that the correlations remained superior to the other techniques, irrespective of the extent of resection or the presence of obstructive airflow limitation (FEV_1/FVC <0.7) [9]. Beccaria and colleagues [8] found similar correlations between predictions based on radionucleotide perfusion scanning and actual postoperative lung function.

Pulmonary quantitative computed tomography scanning

Background

Pulmonary quantitative CT scanning has become an extremely popular modality, given its simplicity, the universal availability of CT scans,

Table 2
Data from a prospective study of 44 pulmonary resection candidates. Correlation coefficients between estimated and measured postoperative values after stratification patients into groups with lobectomy versus pneumonectomy and into groups with normal spirometry versus obstructive airflow limitation

		Lobectomy (n = 34)	Pneumonectomy (n = 10)	FEV1/FVC ≥0.7 (n = 23)	FEV1/FVC <0.7 (n = 21)
FEV_1	CT	0.90	0.88	0.95	0.89
	Q	0.92	0.86	0.92	0.93
	S	0.89	0.47	0.90	0.87
	FS	0.89	0.56	0.87	0.89
	SS	0.88	0.59	0.86	0.89
FVC	CT	0.83	0.81	0.89	0.84
	Q	0.89	0.86	0.90	0.90
	S	0.85	0.49	0.86	0.86
	FS	0.84	0.62	0.82	0.87
	SS	0.85	0.65	0.83	0.88
DL_{CO}, ml/min/mmHg	CT	0.85	0.65	0.77	0.91
	Q	0.86	0.79	0.75	0.93
	S	0.85	0.57	0.76	0.90
	FS	0.85	0.56	0.76	0.91
	SS	0.86	0.56	0.76	0.91
$\dot{V}O_2$ max, ml/kg/min	CT	0.78	0.62	0.67	0.82
	Q	0.88	0.57	0.82	0.89
	S	0.80	0.25	0.64	0.80
	FS	0.77	0.45	0.60	0.82
	SS	0.73	0.42	0.59	0.83

Adapted from Bolliger CT, Guckel C, Engel H, et al. Prediction of functional reserves after lung resection: comparison between quantitative CT, scintigraphy, and anatomy. Respiration 2002;69(6):487; with permission.

and the fact that most lung resection candidates have a preoperative (eg, staging) chest CT scan. Wu and coworkers pioneered [15] the technique in the early 1990s and later refined it following technological advances in the field of CT [16].

Technical aspects

CT scans are performed at full inspiration and viewed with a standard-spatial-frequency reconstruction algorithm and 8-mm collimation with a pitch of 1.25. Semiautomated analyses of the parenchymal views (default range −200 and −1024 H) are then performed in order to identify the "total functional lung volume" (TFLV). The lung parenchyma is outlined from the outer mediastinum and inner chest wall by means of a cursor ball. The next step is to generate three quantitative segments (represented by three different colors) by applying thresholds of greater than −500 H, −500 to −910 H, and less than −910 H by means of commercially available computer programs. Fig. 3 is an example of a quantitative CT scan, where white areas denote emphysema (below −910 H), black areas denote tumor and atelectasis (above −500 H), and gray areas denote the normal lung parenchyma (between −500 and −910 H). The TFLV is then automatically calculated as a volume (the product of color segments areas and section thickness) [16]. The volume of the tumor-bearing lobes or lung is measured in a similar way, and designated the "regional functional lung volume" (RFLV). The CT-predicted FEV_1 values are then calculated as follows: PPO FEV_1 = preoperative FEV_1 × (1−[RFLV/TFLV]) [15]. Similar calculations are performed for PPO FVC.

Correlation of predicted postoperative function based on quantitative computed tomography scanning with actual postoperative lung function

PPO FEV_1 and FVC values as predicted by CT correlate well with actual postoperative measurements. In their landmark study, Wu and coworkers [15] found that, irrespective of the extent of resection, PPO FEV_1 ($r = 0.93$) and PPO FVC ($r = 0.86$) showed statistically significant correlations with postoperative measured values. Subsequent studies by Bolliger and colleagues [9], Wu and colleagues [16], and Ohno and colleagues [17] found comparable

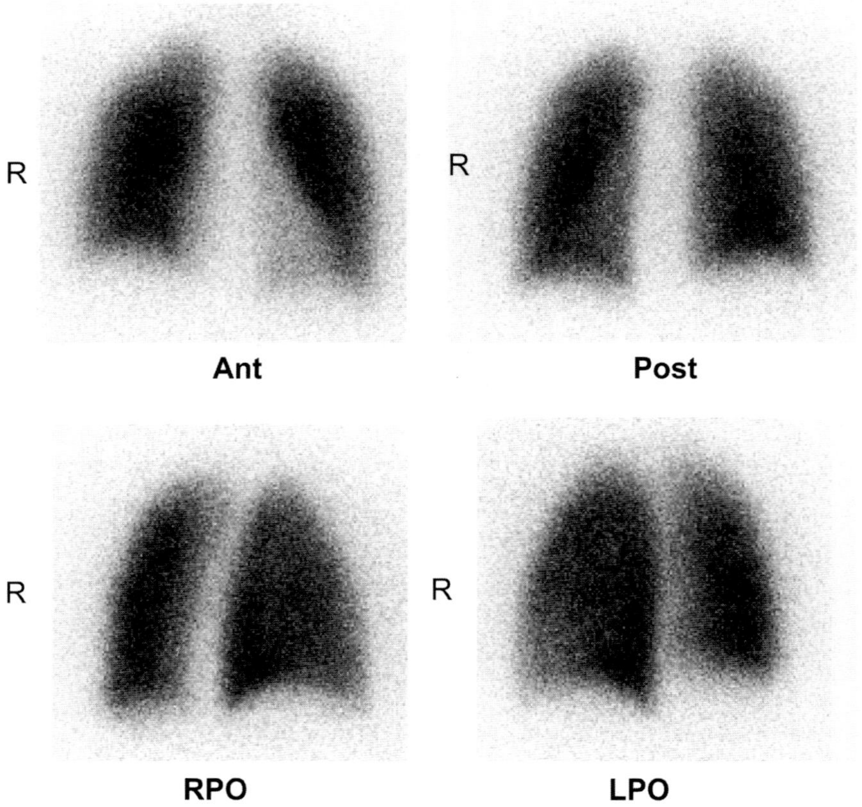

Fig. 2. Radionucleotide perfusion scan. An example of a radionucleotide perfusion scan performed on a patient with normal pulmonary perfusion (technetium-99m SPECT). Quantification is performed by means of a system-integrated, region-ratio program in the anterior (Ant) and posterior (Post) projections for right-left lung quantification (geometric mean), in the left posterior oblique (LPO) projection for left lung lobar quantification and the right posterior oblique (RPO) projection for right lung lobar quantification. (*Courtesy of* Professor Annare Ellmann, Medical Imaging and Clinical Oncology, University of Stellenbosch and Tygerberg Academic Hospital, Cape Town, South Africa.)

correlations. Bolliger and coworkers [9] and Wu and coworkers [16] were also able to show that predictions for FEV_1 and FVC based on quantitative CT were comparable to predictions based on radionucleotide perfusion scanning. Furthermore, both studies also concluded that quantitative CT was more accurate at predicting functional loss after lobectomy ($r = 0.90$) than pneumonectomy ($r = 0.88$). Only Bolliger and colleagues [9] published prospective data on the other parameters frequently used for risk assessment prior to pulmonary resection, namely DL_{CO} and $\dot{V}O_2$ max. They found that CT-derived PPO values for DL_{CO} correlated well ($r = 0.84$) with actual postoperative values, but that CT-derived PPO values for $\dot{V}O_2$ max correlated less well than perfusion scan derived estimates ($r = 0.77$ versus 0.85) [9].

Dynamic contrast-enhanced perfusion magnetic resonance imaging

Background

Three-dimensional (3D) dynamic perfusion MRI is well-established in the evaluation of regional pulmonary perfusion and assessment of physiology and pathophysiology in healthy volunteers, animal models, and patients who have pulmonary vascular disease [17–22]. Until recently, only two small studies [17,21] evaluated the role of this modality in predicting postoperative lung function; however, a large prospective study by Ohno and colleagues published in August 2007 has now firmly established dynamic perfusion MRI as an accurate predictor of postresectional spirometry [18].

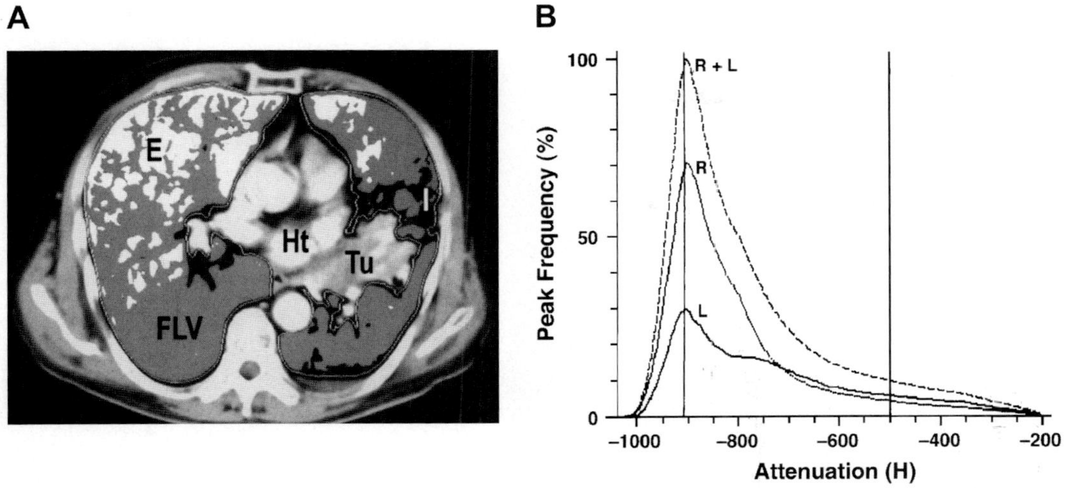

Fig. 3. Pulmonary quantitative CT scan. (*A*) Quantitative CT map shows "functional lung volume" of representative slice. Lung parenchyma was first outlined from mediastinum and chest wall by default range of −200 and −1024 H (white-line contours). Tumor (Tu) was also excluded. After applying dual threshold, three segments in lung parenchyma were generated. White area below −910 H denoted emphysema (E), black area above −500 H denoted infiltration and atelectasis (I), and gray area between −500 and −910 H denoted functional lung volume (FLV). HT, heart. (*B*) Attenuation histogram of quantitative CT integrated from multiple slices encompassing both lungs entirely. Entire lung volume was calculated from area under curve measuring from −1024 to −200 H. Functional lung volume was fractional volume between −500 and −910 H (two vertical lines). Functional lung volume of left lung was 1363 mL; functional lung volume of right lung was 2292 mL. Left/right ratio of functional lung volume was 35% versus 65%. Quantitative CT–FEV_1 loss was 35%. L, left lung; R, right lung; R + L, combination. (*From* Wu MT, Pan HB, Chiang AA, et al. Prediction of postoperative lung function in patients with lung cancer: comparison of quantitative CT with perfusion scintigraphy. Am J Roentgenol 2002;178(3):668; with permission.)

Technical aspects

Dynamic perfusion MRI studies are performed on a 1.5-T scanner using a phased array coil. The studies are acquired with a 3D radiofrequency spoiled gradient-echo sequence (Fig. 4). A 100-mm, 10-partition 3D slab thickness should be used with a contiguous slice in the coronal plane and a left-to-right, phase-encoded direction [17,18]. A bolus of 3–5 mL of gadopentetate dimeglumine is administered with an automatic infusion system prior to the scan. Patients are then instructed to hold their breath for 25 seconds, during which time 25 images are obtained.

Analyzing and interpreting the data acquired by means of dynamic contrast-enhanced perfusion MRI requires some degree of expertise as well as appropriate computer software. Signal intensity–time course curves are generated (after administration of contrast) by measurement of the signal intensity in regions of interest (ROIs) delineated in the right upper, right middle, right lower, left upper, left middle, and left lower lung fields in every slice. Large vessels and pulmonary arteries are excluded from the ROIs. For extraction of quantitative indices, the signal intensity–time course curves are fitted to a gamma variate function with a validated equation [17,21]. From the gamma variate function, a further validated equation is used to calculate the apparent mean transit time as the first moment on the MRI signal intensity–time course curve. Regional pulmonary blood volume is then calculated from the area of the MRI signal intensity–time course curve for a given ROI. According to the central volume principle, regional blood flow in each ROI is then determined by dividing pulmonary blood volume by mean transit time [17,20]. The ROI blood flow value is normalized to the integrated arterial input function from the main trunk of the pulmonary artery [17,20]. A special formula is subsequently used to determine regional perfusion in a lung field on dynamic contrast-enhanced perfusion MRI (blood flow in an ROI expressed as a percentage) in order to predict postoperative lung function. Finally, PPO FEV_1 is derived as follows: PPO FEV_1 (perfusion MRI) = FEV_1 × (1−[percentage of perfusion resected lobe or

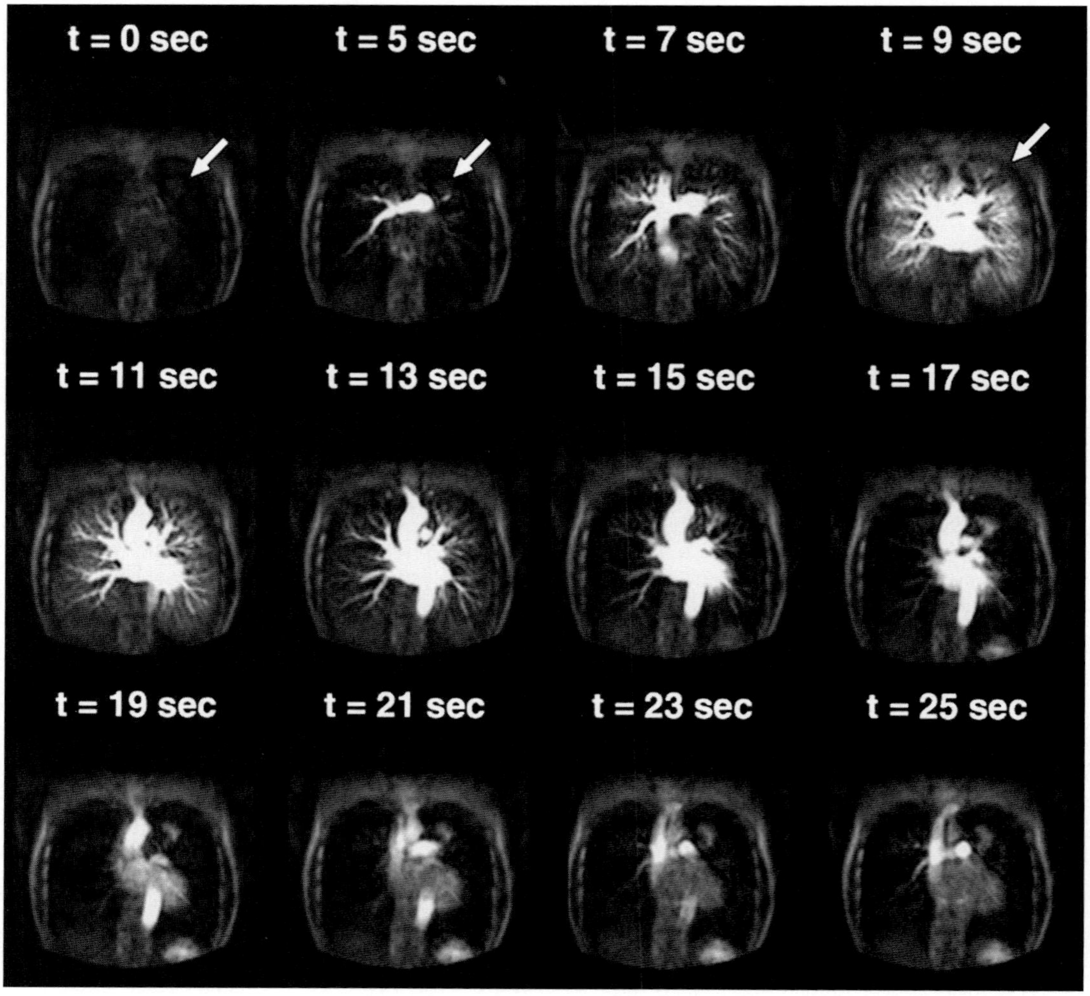

Fig. 4. Dynamic perfusion MRI. A dynamic perfusion MRI of a 63-year-old man with adenocarcinoma in upper lobe of left lung. The images show heterogeneous but well-enhanced pulmonary parenchyma at 5 and 13 seconds in portions of lungs not affected by lung cancer (*arrows*). Lung cancer also is enhanced after 13 seconds. (*From* Ohno Y, Koyama H, Nogami M, et al. Postoperative lung function in lung cancer patients: comparative analysis of predictive capability of MRI, CT, and SPECT. Am J Roentgenol. 2007;189(2):404; with permission.)

lung/100]). A detailed discussion on technical aspects, including the formulae required, can be found in reference [18].

Correlation of predicted postoperative function based on dynamic perfusion magnetic resonance imaging with actual postoperative lung function

Ohno and colleagues' [18] study is one of the largest prospective studies in the field of predicted postoperative lung functions. They compared dynamic perfusion MRI's ability to predict post-operative FEV_1 with that of CT and SPECT. The actual postoperative FEV_1 had stronger correlation with the PPO FEV_1 predicted from perfusion MRI ($r = 0.87$) and quantitative CT ($r = 0.88$) than with postoperative FEV1 predicted from SPECT ($r = 0.83$). The limits of agreement between the actual postoperative FEV_1 and postoperative FEV_1 predicted from perfusion MRI (5.3% ± 11.8%) were smaller than the values for postoperative FEV_1 predicted from perfusion SPECT (5.1% ± 14.0%), and were almost equal to the values for postoperative FEV_1 predicted from quantitative CT (5.0% ± 11.6%). The study authors concluded that dynamic perfusion MRI was more accurate in the prediction of the postoperative lung function than perfusion SPECT, and possibly at least as accurate as quantitative CT. Of note is the fact that other parameters of lung function (most notably DL_{CO} and $\dot{V}O_2$ max) were not assessed.

Vibration response imaging

A novel way to assess regional lung function was described in the late 1990s. Vibration response imaging (VRI) makes use of piezoelectric contact sensors to detect turbulent air and vibrations within the lungs and airways that are transmitted to the skin [23,24]. Provisional results show that VRI energy correlates with the regional ventilation ($r = 0.70$) and perfusion ($r = 0.65$) when compared with standard ventilation and perfusion radionucleotide scanning; however, no prospective studies have been published on PPO lung functions following pulmonary resection. If validated, this technique may become an attractive alternative because it is completely noninvasive.

A practical approach to the assessment of regional lung function prior to pulmonary resection

Patients who have preserved pulmonary functions do not benefit from the assessment of regional lung function prior to lung resection [1–4]. Patients who have an FEV_1 or a DL_{CO} of less than 80% of predicted warrant a formal exercise test, and if their exercise capacity is impaired ($\dot{V}O_2$ max not more than 20 mL/kg/min or 75% of predicted), need calculations of the PPO values of the before-mentioned parameters (see Fig. 1) [1–4]. There are centers where split studies are performed prior to formal exercise tests, but the cost effectiveness of this approach has been questioned, because exercise tests are cheap and noninvasive [1–4].

Estimations of PPO lung function based on anatomical calculations are by far the simplest way of predicting postresectional lung function: the number of functional segments that are due for resection is subtracted from the total number of functional segments, and this value is divided by the total number of functional segments to give a fraction (see equations above) [3,9]. Although these calculations are less accurate than other techniques, they remain useful screening tools because they err on the side of safety. Anatomical estimations have been shown in prospective studies to overestimate functional loss, because there may be minimal loss after removal of destroyed, collapsed, or tumor-bearing lung parenchyma [3,9]. A sensible approach, therefore, would be to perform anatomical calculations in each pulmonary resection candidate requiring assessment of PPO lung function, and to reserve the more complex techniques for the borderline or apparently inoperable cases.

Choosing the next appropriate investigation is more complex. Recent advances in radiology with regards to quantitative CT scanning and dynamic contrast-enhanced perfusion MRI have certainly challenged radionucleotide perfusion scanning as the gold standard for the assessment of regional lung function [16–18]. Comparing prospective data from different studies is, however, extremely challenging, given variations in study protocols and local expertise and equipment. Furthermore, most recent studies only assessed the ability of the different modalities to predict postoperative FEV_1. It should be kept in mind that both PPO DL_{CO} and PPO $\dot{V}O_2$ max predict postoperative complications [2–4], and that quantitative CT scanning, for example, fared less well at predicting PPO $\dot{V}O_2$ max than PPO FEV_1, at least in one study [9].

A further interesting observation is the fact that local expertise and experience dictated which of the three basic techniques was superior at predicting PPO FEV in prospective studies: radionucleotide perfusion scanning in the case of Bolliger and colleagues [9], quantitative CT scanning in the case of Wu and colleagues [16] or dynamic contrast-enhanced perfusion MRI as shown by Ohno and colleagues [18].

In conclusion, clinicians are advised to perform anatomical calculations on all patients who require preoperative estimation of postoperative lung function. Patients who require further evaluation (often because of borderline or suspected high-risk postoperative function) will require one of three special investigations, namely radionucleotide perfusion scanning, quantitative CT scanning, or dynamic contrast-enhanced perfusion MRI. Current evidence suggests that all three techniques perform comparatively well at predicting postoperative FEV_1. Cost, local expertise and availability, and the need to predict PPO $\dot{V}O_2$ max should dictate the clinician's choice when requesting an assessment of regional lung function. Staging CT scans are invariably performed preoperatively on practically all lung cancer patients. Quantitative CT scanning is therefore arguably the investigation of choice with regards to the prediction of postoperative function, because it is well-validated [9,16–18], generally available, and relatively cheap (requires only extra software, time, and some expertise).

Some unanswered questions remain. Lung volume reduction surgery for end-stage emphysema has, to an extent, redefined the limits of lung resection. These patients have traditionally been excluded from studies on the predictive capability of SPECT, CT, or MRI, and the general tolerability of the procedure confirms the conservative nature of the current thresholds and the fact that removal of the most diseased regions may permit better function of other regions. It remains to be determined whether the formal assessment of regional lung function alters the risk stratification of patients who undergo tumor resection in conjunction with lung volume reduction surgery, although upper lobe predominance of the emphysematous changes have been associated with a more favorable outcome [25].

References

[1] Bolliger CT. Evaluation of operability before lung resection. Curr Opin Pulm Med 2003;9:321–6.

[2] Bolliger CT, Kendal R, Koegelenberg CF. Preoperative assessment for lung cancer surgery. Curr Opin Pulm Med 2005;11(4):301–6.

[3] Bolliger CT, Perruchoud AP. Functional evaluation of the lung resection candidate. Eur Respir J 1998; 11:198–212.

[4] Wyser C, Stulz P, Soler M, et al. Prospective evaluation of an algorithm for the functional assessment of lung resection candidates. Am J Respir Crit Care Med 1999;159:1450–6.

[5] Jacobaeus HC, Frenckner P, Björkman S. Some attempts at determining the volume and function of each lung separately. Acta Med Scand 1932;79: 174–215.

[6] Carlens E. A new flexible double-lumen catheter for bronchospirometry. J Thorac Surg 1949;18:742–6.

[7] Pierce RJ, Copland JM, Sharpe K, et al. Preoperative risk evaluation for lung cancer resection: predicted postoperative product as a predictor of surgical mortality. Am J Respir Crit Care Med 1994;150:947–55.

[8] Beccaria M, Corsico A, Fulgonie P, et al. Lung cancer resection. The prediction of postsurgical outcomes should include long-term functional results. Chest 2001;120:37–42.

[9] Bolliger CT, Guckel C, Engel H, et al. Prediction of functional reserves after lung resection: comparison between quantitative computed tomography, scintigraphy, and anatomy. Respiration 2002;69(6): 482–9.

[10] Nakahara K, Monden Y, Ohno K, et al. A method for predicting postoperative lung function and its relation to postoperative complications in patients with lung cancer. Ann Thorac Surg 1985;39:260–5.

[11] Knipping HW, Bolt W, Valentin H, et al. Eine neue Methode zur Prüfung der Herz-und Lungenfunktion. Dtsch Med Wochenschr 1955;80:1146–7 [in German].

[12] Kristersson S, Lindell S-E, Svanberg L. Prediction of pulmonary function loss due to pneumonectomy using 133Xe-radiospirometry. Chest 1972;62: 694–8.

[13] Olsen GN, Block AJ, Tobias JA. Prediction of postpneumonectomy pulmonary function using quantitative macroaggregate lung scanning. Chest 1974; 66:13–6.

[14] Markos J, Mullan BP, Hillman DR, et al. Preoperative assessment as a predictor of mortality and morbidity after lung resection. Am Rev Respir Dis 1989; 139:902–10.

[15] Wu MT, Chang JM, Chiang AA, et al. Use of quantitative CT to predict postoperative lung function in patients with lung cancer. Radiology 1994;191: 257–62.

[16] Wu MT, Pan HB, Chiang AA, et al. Prediction of postoperative lung function in patients with lung cancer: comparison of quantitative CT with perfusion scintigraphy. Am J Roentgenol 2002;178: 667–72.

[17] Ohno Y, Hatabu H, Higashino T, et al. Dynamic perfusion MRI versus perfusion scintigraphy: prediction of postoperative lung function in patients with lung cancer. Am J Roentgenol 2004;182(1): 73–8.

[18] Ohno Y, Koyama H, Nogami M, et al. Postoperative lung function in lung cancer patients: comparative analysis of predictive capability of MRI, CT, and SPECT. Am J Roentgenol 2007;189(2): 400–8.

[19] Hatabu H, Gaa J, Kim D, et al. Pulmonary perfusion: qualitative assessment with dynamic contrast-enhanced MRI using ultrashort TE and inversion recovery turbo FLASH. Magn Reson Med 1996; 36:503–8.

[20] Levin DL, Chen Q, Zhang M, et al. Evaluation of regional pulmonary perfusion using ultrafast magnetic resonance imaging. Magn Reson Med 2001; 46:166–71.

[21] Iwasawa T, Saito K, Ogawa N, et al. Prediction of postoperative pulmonary function using perfusion magnetic resonance imaging of the lung. J Magn Reson Imaging 2002;15:685–92.

[22] Ohno Y, Hatabu H, Murase K, et al. Quantitative assessment of regional pulmonary perfusion in the entire lung using three-dimensional ultrafast dynamic contrast-enhanced magnetic resonance

imaging: preliminary experience in 40 subjects. J Magn Reson Imaging 2004;20:353–65.
[23] Pasterkamp H, Kraman SS, Wodicka GR. Respiratory sounds. Advances beyond the stethoscope. Am J Respir Crit Care Med 1997;156:974–87.
[24] Dellinger RP, Parrillo JE, Kushnir A, et al. Dynamic visualization of lung sounds with a vibration response device: a case series. Respiration 2007; [Epub ahead of print].
[25] National Emphysema Treatment Trial Research Group. A randomized trial comparing lung-volume reduction surgery with medical therapy for severe emphysema. N Engl J Med 2003;348: 2059–73.

ELSEVIER
SAUNDERS

Thorac Surg Clin 18 (2008) 31–37

THORACIC
SURGERY
CLINICS

Future Trends in Preoperative Evaluation

Gonzalo Varela, MD, PhD, FETCS*, Nuria M. Novoa, MD, PhD

Service of Thoracic Surgery, Salamanca University Hospital, Paseo San Vicente 58-182, Salamanca, Spain

Preoperative evaluation before major thoracic procedures is aimed at classifying patients according to their probability of adverse postoperative outcomes and the estimated effectiveness of the surgical procedure. Operative mortality is the most relevant outcome but its modern occurrence is not high and it can be considered a rare event. According to recent publications, the mortality of a standard lobectomy is around 2% [1–3] and the rate for standard pneumonectomy is under 5% [1–3]. Because mortality is a rather infrequent event, large databases are required to increase the predictive power of mathematical models. Even using the results of such databases, caution is required interpreting the prediction of a risk model in the case of an individual patient [1]. First, large databases lack homogeneity not only in the population under analysis but also in the specific perioperative procedures. Generalization of published results to a different population can be inaccurate because it has been shown that the percentage of adverse events published by large academic centers is lower than what can be found reviewing the activity of centers outside the academic surroundings [4], despite the fact that teaching hospitals perform more complex and high-risk procedures [5].

The limitations of currently available multifactorial indexes have been recently reviewed [6]. The first comes from the existing cut-points of pulmonary volumes under which patients are not operated. Estimated postoperative values of pulmonary volumes, mainly forced expiratory volume in 1 second (FEV_1), are not reliable predictors of complications in patients with chronic obstructive pulmonary disease (COPD), because these patients can experience a paradoxical improvement of immediate postoperative pulmonary function [7]. Pulmonary volumes 3 to 6 months after surgery can be accurately calculated [8], but they are unable to predict what is going to happen in the immediate postoperative period when most of the complications are developed [9]. Finally, the restriction of diffusing capacity of lung for carbon monoxide (DLCO) measurement or exercise tests only to patients with low pulmonary volumes, according to the most used guidelines [10,11], limits its predictive value [[illegible]].

It has been recently published that Thoracoscore multifactor index is highly accurate (C-index >0.8) for early [12] and mid term mortality in patients undergoing thoracic surgery [13]. To develop the Thoracoscore system, the authors prospectively collected data from more than 15,000 patients who underwent thoracic procedures. To build up and test the model, they included many different clinical variables, such as the priority of the surgical procedure (including emergency procedures) or the performance status of the patient (including cases ≥3 of the World Health Organization). Although the performance of the model both in the training and validation subsets of cases was superior to that observed in other models, it is not applicable to cancer patients scheduled for lung resection because lung resection for cancer is rarely performed as an emergency and patients with low performance status are excluded from this kind of surgery.

Selecting relevant and frequent outcomes

In most papers dealing with preoperative evaluation for lung resection, operative mortality or cardiorespiratory morbidity is selected as target outcome. Mortality is the worst adverse event of surgery, whereas postoperative morbidity is

* Corresponding author.
E-mail address: gvs@usal.es (G. Varela).

1547-4127/08/$ - see front matter
doi:10.1016/j.thorsurg.2007.10.006

a relevant outcome from the surgeon's side but, in some cases, it is not regarded as such from the patient's perspective. In a published investigation [14], outcomes reflecting physical debility (need of continuous assistance, permanent placement in a nursing home, existence limited to bed-to-chair activity, and so forth) were considered the worst (after death) by a series of patients being evaluated for lung resection. Outcomes of lung resection related to quality of life (QOL) are not usually investigated. In a recent paper by Brunelli and colleagues [15] the authors conclude that postoperative QOL measures did not correlate with postoperative pulmonary volumes and exercise performance. QOL parameters should be considered during the preoperative evaluation process, keeping in mind that patients undergoing lung resection have a preoperative impairment of their QOL parameters, compared with the general population [15,16] and transient adverse effects of surgery on QOL should not be regarded as contraindications for lung resection [16].

Besides introducing QOL parameters, the concept of surgical mortality should be reviewed. It has been suggested that mortality risk 1 year after operation could be a meaningful outcome, both from the surgeon's and from the patient's perspectives [17]. In a large database of patients from the UK Heart Valve Registry, 30-day mortality represented only 56% of 1-year mortality. The authors have not found comparable data related to lung resection but it can be expected that delayed mortality after resection for lung cancer should be superior to 30-day, even if tumor-related mortality is excluded. The reason is that a high rate of cases operated on for lung cancer have some degree of COPD and, as was published by Sekine and colleagues [18], respiratory failure is a major cause of non–cancer-related death in COPD operated patients.

Prediction of postoperative pulmonary volumes

Estimation of postoperative FEV_1% (ppo-FEV_1%) is a frequently used criterion to define functional operability in patients undergoing lung resection [11] because low ppoFEV_1% value correlates with the occurrence of postoperative morbidity and mortality as a single predictor [19] or in combination with other variables [1]. In a previous paper [20], it was shown that current methods of prediction of postoperative FEV_1 greatly underestimated the real functional loss in the immediate postoperative period (Fig. 1). Postoperative cardiorespiratory complications are more related to FEV_1 measured in the first postoperative day than to ppoFEV_1 value [9]. According to this finding, a mathematical model was suggested to predict early FEV_1 after lobectomy [21]. In a preliminary series of operated cases receiving correct postoperative analgesia, a good correlation was obtained between values of predicted FEV_1 and observed the first day after major lung resection (Fig. 2), and although the model is not ready for patient selection, it is being tested as a new tool for risk stratification.

Recently, several studies have demonstrated minimal loss or even improvement in pulmonary function after lobectomy in COPD patients [22–29]. This effect can also be found in the early postoperative period at 1 week [21] or the day after the operation [6]. The evidence that some degree of lung-volume reduction effect takes place in the early postoperative period could in the future modify currently accepted FEV_1 and ppoFEV_1 cut-points for lobectomy.

Routine indication of diffusing capacity of lung for carbon monoxide measurement and exercise tests

As has recently been pointed out [6], DLCO and exercise tests are frequently indicated in the evaluation of candidates for lung resection only after the finding of a low ppoFEV_1 value. In some published papers [30], it is assumed that a ppoFEV_1 greater than 40% accurately identifies patients not requiring additional tests because of low risk of postoperative and long-term pulmonary insufficiency. This practice is in contradiction with prospectively tested guidelines [31]. In a paper by Brunelli and colleagues [32], DLCO was routinely performed in all surgical candidates finding that even in subjects with otherwise apparently normal pulmonary function, the reduction of the diffusion capacity was highly predictive of postoperative morbidity. This and other evidences suggest that DLCO should be preoperatively investigated as a routine before lung resection and this recommendation becomes mandatory in patients being considered for surgical therapy after induction chemotherapy because of the impairment of DLCO values secondary to pulmonary toxicity [33].

The prognostic significance of DLCO could be increased if the test is performed after standardized exercise. As published by Wang and colleagues [34], measuring DLCO at rest does not evaluate the capacity of the lung to increase

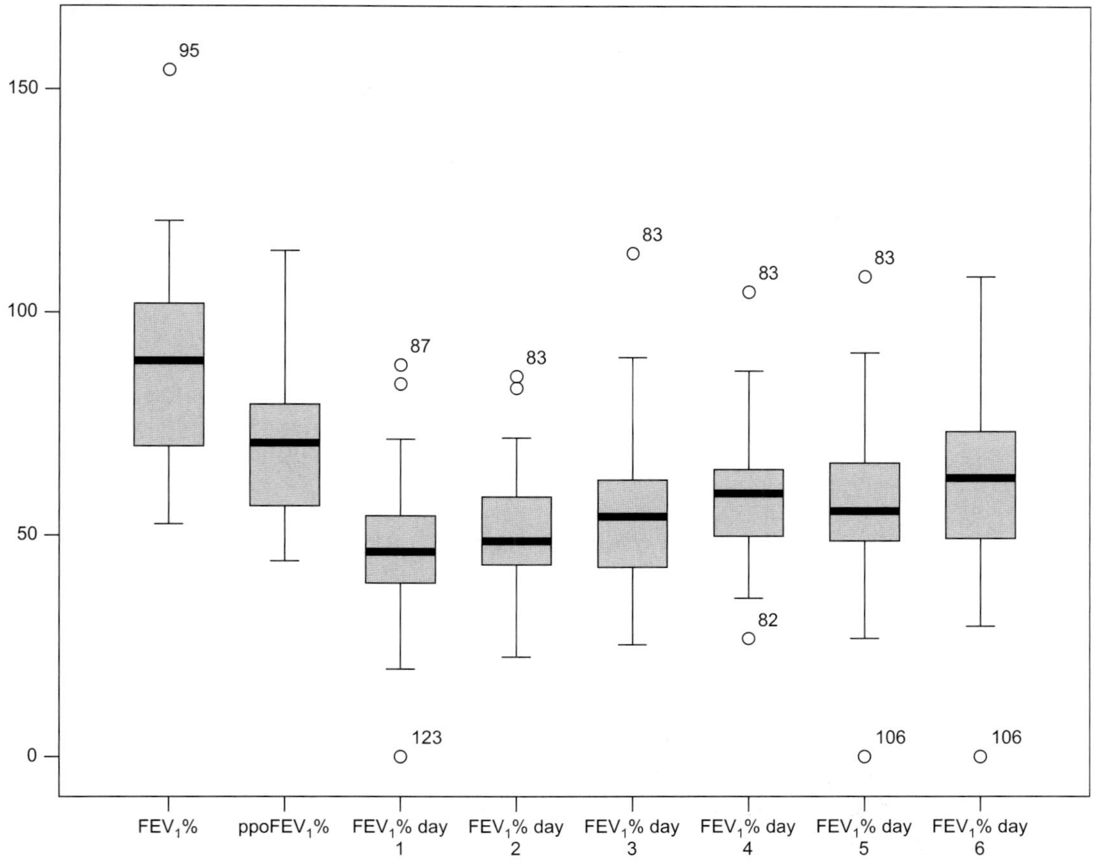

Fig. 1. Comparison of preoperative FEV_1%, ppoFEV_1% and measured postoperative FEV_1% on postoperative days 1 to 6. (*From* Varela G, Brunelli A, Rocco G, et al. Predicted versus observed FEV_1 in the immediate postoperative period after pulmonary lobectomy. Eur J Cardiothorac Surg 2006;30:644–8; with permission.)

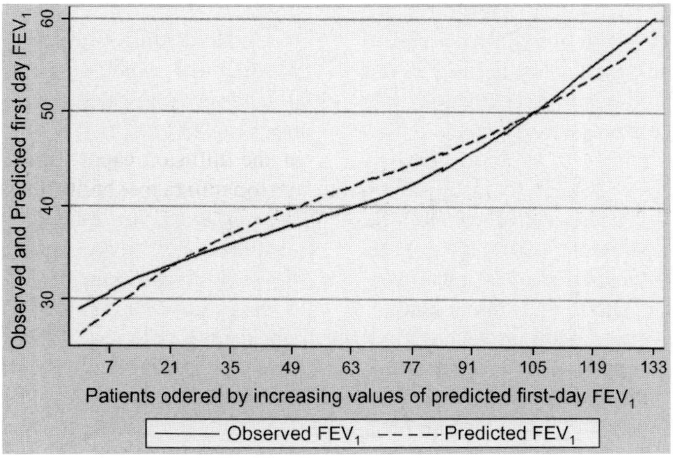

Fig. 2. Predicted versus observed FEV_1 the first day after major pulmonary resection in a series of 272 cases. (*From* Brunelli A, Varela G, Rocco G, et al. A model to predict the immediate postoperative FEV1 following major lung resections. Eur J Cardio Thorac Surg 2007;32:783–6; with permission.)

oxygen diffusion during exercise. These investigators have found that patients without an increase of at least 10% in their DLCO after submaximal exercise (compared with rest values) are prone to postoperative complications. During exercise, the lung experiences an increase in ventilation, oxygen uptake, carbon dioxide output, and blood flow similar to the one observed during the postoperative period after lung resection. A single test can be used to assess the physiologic response after surgery and it is hypothesized that those patients unable to perform adequately on exercise testing may similarly to do so in response to surgical stress or adverse postoperative events, and performance on exercise testing should be better correlated to surgical outcome than other parameters.

Preoperative exercise tests require high-technology equipment and are expensive. Consequently, they are indicated in a small percentage of cases, mostly after predicting postoperative pulmonary volumes or DLCO.

Less sophisticated tests should be evaluated in large series of nonbiased cases as predictors of poor postoperative outcome. Among simple tests, stair climbing is one of the most reliable. The altitude reached at the stair climbing test correlates with postoperative outcome according to Girish and colleagues [35] and Brunelli and colleagues [36]. In the latter article [36], Vo_2max was also estimated from the maximal work during the test. They found no differences in Vo_2max between patients with $ppoFEV_1$ under 40% and those having greater than or equal to 40%. Interestingly, 17 cases with a $ppoFEV_1$ under 40% were operated on according to their better performance on the exercise test with no mortality and standard morbidity. Patients unable to perform a preoperative maximal exercise test because of incapacitating comorbidities had an increased risk of mortality after major lung resection.

Other simple tests related to exercise capacity could be prospectively evaluated to facilitate its widespread use in the preoperative evaluation, because most cases operated on for lung cancer are elderly and COPD patients. It has been demonstrated that in COPD, the impairment of the oxidative capacity of striated muscle is related to the fast increase of blood lactate during exercise [37] along with a delayed clearance from the circulation. Lack of training and sedentary habits, which can be quantified independently of patient's age [38], have been identified as one of the reasons for lactate increase [39]. Elderly patients suffer a decrease of capillary density in COPD cases [37] and a relevant decrease of blood flow through the lower extremities, however, which is neither dependent on COPD nor on exercise habits [40]. Finally, in some COPD cases, even in patients with mild or moderate disease, a decrease of muscle endurance has been demonstrated [41]. All these factors can be unveiled during simple exercise tests and can be correlated to postoperative outcome. It can also be hypothesized that the degree of a patient's daily activity before surgery can be used as a reliable parameter to estimate the risk of lung resection. In a recent paper by Manini and colleagues [42], daily living energy expenditure was assessed in 302 healthy older adults (age range, 70–82 years) finding that energy expenditure was strongly associated with lower risk of mortality. Another simple useful parameter to estimate surgical risk is the evaluation of preoperative daily activity by means of a nonexpensive commercially available pedometer. According to a report published some years ago [43], motion detectors are useful to measure daily activity related to physiologic impairment caused by COPD and other diseases. The amount and intensity of daily physical activity is closely related to health and mortality. Subjective methods (eg, questionnaires and dyspnea indexes) have been found to be less accurate to evaluate the amount of daily physical activity performed than motion sensors [44], and the addition of such simple nonexpensive parameters to preoperative evaluation could result in better knowledge of the patient's performance status.

Mathematical improvements

Understanding statistics is basic to understanding the validity of a clinical investigation [45]. Nevertheless, designing accurate methods for modeling surgical risk is not a basic skill for surgeons. Many multi-institutional databases contain a large number of records and variables, whereas relevant events are difficult to predict because of low prevalence. Inviting experts in biologic modeling to join clinicians to form multidisciplinary investigation teams improves the validity of the conclusions and the design of future projects. Finding good experimental designs to predict cardiorespiratory morbidity or mortality after lung resection can decrease the number of cases needed to construct a valid model [46]. Classification trees are powerful analytical tools that produce understandable results as tree diagrams and can be useful for a better understanding of the final results

[9]. Although logistic regression assumes the linearity and independence of predictors, classification trees can discover the interaction among predictors that do not show strong marginal effects [9]. Nevertheless, advanced predictive mathematical models are beyond the scope of surgical education and are better performed by specially trained professionals.

Summary

Preoperative evaluation before lung resection has been frequently addressed in modern medical literature. Actual or predicted pulmonary volumes are considered relevant to predict the risk of surgery. Nevertheless, ppoFEV_1 underestimates the real functional loss in the immediate postoperative period when most of the complications occur. Not all patients, however, have comparable functional changes after lobectomy. Minimal impairment or even improvements have been demonstrated in COPD cases after lobectomy. Efforts should be directed to an accurate prediction of the immediate postoperative pulmonary volumes for a better evaluation of high-risk patients caused by respiratory impairment.

Future developments are needed on the role of measuring preoperative DLCO and how to evaluate a patient's general cardiorespiratory status. Evidence underlines the relevance of routine evaluation of preoperative DLCO at rest or, better, during exercise for a thorough assessment of patient's capability to adapt to a stressful situation (Fig. 3). Only by improving knowledge about the general condition of the patient, can one assess the physiologic response to surgery. Widespread use of sophisticated or simple exercise tests and

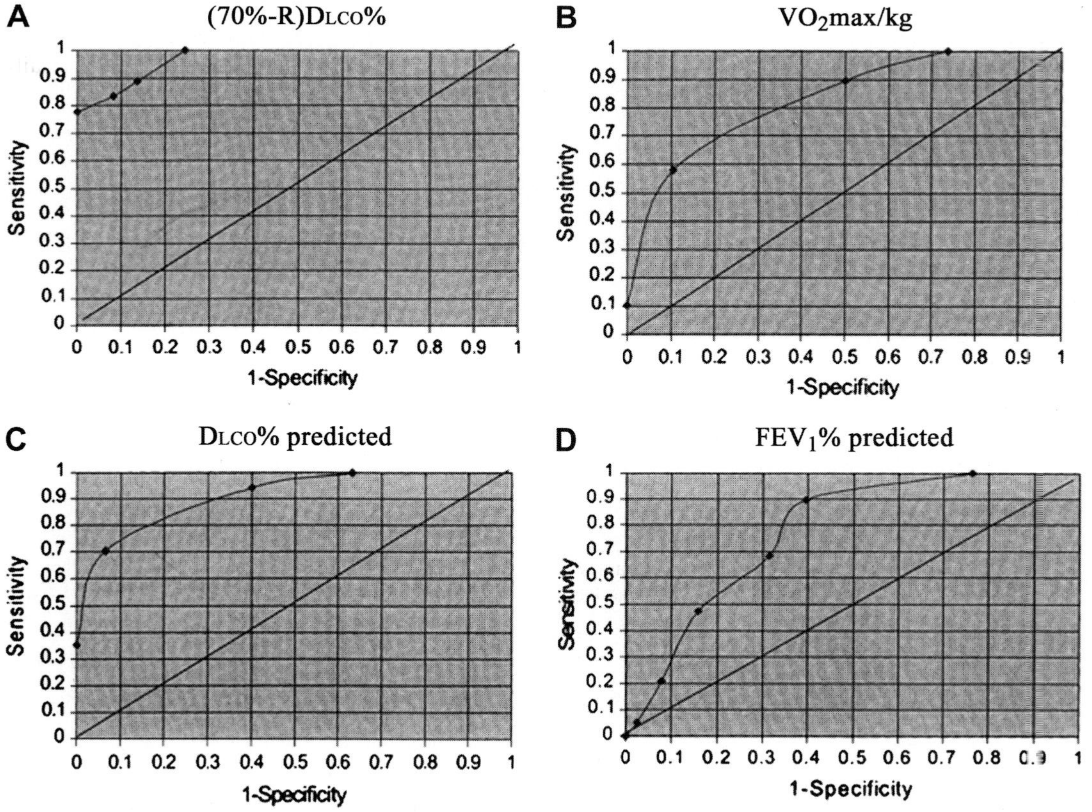

Fig. 3. (*A–D*) ROC curves showing the predictive performance of different parameters in a series of patients operated on for lung carcinoma. The most predictive parameter is seen in *A*: increase in diffusing capacity of lung for carbon monoxide (DLCO) from rest to 70% of maximal workload expressed as a percent of the predicted DLCO at rest. (*From* Wang JS, Abboud RT, Evans KG, et al. Role of CO diffusing capacity during exercise in the preoperative evaluation for lung resection. Am J Respir Crit Care Med 2000;162:1435–44; with permission.)

measurements of daily activity using motion detectors can identify high-risk patients with otherwise acceptable pulmonary volumes.

Another suggested investigation issue is to develop different relevant outcome parameters, not only from the surgeon's point of view but also from the patient's perspective, such as postoperative QOL-related variables or delayed outcomes. Finally, multidisciplinary investigation teams, including experts in mathematical modeling, are essential to improve the quality and validity of the developed models.

Although knowledge about perioperative physiologic changes has increased, clinicians are still far from finding a way to put all this knowledge down and make it applicable for an individual patient. Multicentric cooperation and evaluation of large prospectively recorded databases are essential to develop evidence-based clinical guidelines on preoperative evaluation.

References

[1] Berrisford R, Brunelli A, Rocco G, et al. The European Thoracic Surgery Database project: modelling the risk of in-hospital death following lung resection. Eur J Cardiothorac Surg 2005;28:306–11.

[2] Memtsoudis SG, Besculides MC, Zellos L, et al. Trends in lung surgery: United States 1988 to 2002. Chest 2006;130:1462–70.

[3] Wada H, Nakamura T, Nakamoto K, et al. Thirty-day operative mortality for thoracotomy in lung cancer. J Thorac Cardiovasc Surg 1998;115:70–3.

[4] Romano PS, Mark DH. Patient and hospital characteristics related to in-hospital mortality after lung cancer resection. Chest 1992;101:1332–7.

[5] Khuri SF, Najjar SF, Daley J, et al. Comparison of surgical outcomes between teaching and non-teaching hospitals in the Department of Veterans Affairs. Ann Surg 2001;234:370–82.

[6] Brunelli A, Rocco G, Varela G. Predictive ability of preoperative indices for major pulmonary surgery. Thorac Surg Clin 2007;17:329–36.

[7] Varela G, Brunelli A, Rocco G, et al. Evidence of lower alteration of expiratory volume in patients with airflow limitation in the immediate period after lobectomy. Ann Thorac Surg 2007;84:417–22.

[8] Bolliger CT, Wyser C, Roser H, et al. Lung scanning and exercise testing for the prediction of postoperative performance in lung resection candidates at increased risk for complications. Chest 1995;108: 341–8.

[9] Varela G, Brunelli A, Rocco G, et al. Measured FEV1 in the first postoperative day, and not ppo-FEV1, is the best predictor of cardio-respiratory morbidity after lung resection. Eur J Cardiothorac Surg 2007;31:518–21.

[10] British Thoracic Society, Society of Cardiothoracic Surgeons of Great Britian, Ireland Working Party. BTS guidelines: guidelines on the selection of patients with lung cancer for surgery. Thorax 2001; 56:89–108.

[11] Beckles MA, Spiro SG, Colice GL, et al. The physiologic evaluation of patients with lung cancer being considered for resectional surgery. Chest 2003;123 (1 Suppl):105S–14S.

[12] Falcoz PE, Conti M, Brouchet L, et al. The thoracic surgery scoring system (Thoracoscore): risk model for in-hospital death in 15,183 patients requiring thoracic surgery. J Thorac Cardiovasc Surg 2007; 133:325–32.

[13] Chamogeorgakis TP, Connery CP, Bhora F, et al. Thoracoscore predicts midterm mortality in patients undergoing thoracic surgery. J Thorac Cardiovasc Surg 2007;134:883–7.

[14] Cykert S. Risk acceptance and risk aversion: patients' perspectives on lung surgery. Thorac Surg Clin 2004;14:287–93.

[15] Brunelli A, Socci L, Refai M, et al. Quality of life before and after major lung resection for lung cancer: a prospective follow-up analysis. Ann Thorac Surg 2007;84:410–6.

[16] McManus K. Concerns of poor quality of life should not deprive patients of the opportunity of curative surgery. Thorax 2003;58:189.

[17] Edwards MB, Taylor KM. Is 30-day mortality an adequate outcome statistic for patients considering heart valve replacement? Ann Thorac Surg 2003; 76:482–5.

[18] Sekine Y, Behnia M, Fujisawa T. Impact of COPD on pulmonary complications and on long-term survival of patients undergoing surgery for NSCLC. Lung Cancer 2002;37:95–101.

[19] Kearney DJ, Lee TH, Reilly JJ, et al. Assessment of operative risk in patients undergoing lung resection: importance of predicted pulmonary function. Chest 1994;105:753–9.

[20] Varela G, Brunelli A, Rocco G, et al. Predicted versus observed FEV1 in the immediate postoperative period after pulmonary lobectomy. Eur J Cardiothorac Surg 2006;30:644–8.

[21] Brunelli A, Varela G, Rocco G, et al. A model to predict the immediate postoperative FEV1 following major lung resections. Eur J Cardiothorac Surg 2007; doi:10.1016/j.ejcts.2007.07.014.

[22] Korst RJ, Ginsberg RJ, Ailawadi M, et al. Lobectomy improves ventilatory function in selected patients with severe COPD. Ann Thorac Surg 1998;66:898–902.

[23] Carretta A, Zannini P, Puglisi A, et al. Improvement of pulmonary function after lobectomy for non-small cell lung cancer in emphysematous patients. Eur J Cardiothorac Surg 1999;15:602–7.

[24] Santambrogio L, Nosotti M, Baisi A, et al. Pulmonary lobectomy for lung cancer: a prospective study to compare patients with forced expiratory volume

in 1 s more or less than 80% of predicted. Eur J Cardiothorac Surg 2001;20:684–7.

[25] Edwards JG, Duthie DJ, Waller DA. Lobar volume reduction surgery: a method of increasing the lung cancer resection rate in patients with emphysema. Thorax 2001;56:791–5.

[26] Sekine Y, Iwata T, Chiyo M, et al. Minimal alteration of pulmonary function after lobectomy in lung cancer patients with chronic obstructive pulmonary disease. Ann Thorac Surg 2003;76: 356–61.

[27] Baldi S, Ruffini E, Harari S, et al. Does lobectomy for lung cancer in patients with chronic obstructive pulmonary disease affect lung function? A multicenter national study. J Thorac Cardiovasc Surg 2005; 130:1616–22.

[28] Brunelli A, Xiume F, Refai M, et al. Evaluation of expiratory volume, diffusion capacity, and exercise tolerance following major lung resection: a prospective follow-up analysis. Chest 2007;131: 141–7.

[29] Brunelli A, Refai M, Salati M, et al. Predicted versus observed FEV1 and DLCO after major lung resection: a prospective evaluation at different postoperative periods. Ann Thorac Surg 2007;83:1134–9.

[30] Beccaria M, Corsico A, Fulgoni P, et al. Lung cancer resection: the prediction of postsurgical outcomes should include long-term functional results. Chest 2001;120:37–42.

[31] Wyser C, Stulz P, Soler M, et al. Prospective evaluation of an algorithm for the functional assessment of lung resection candidates. Am J Respir Crit Care Med 1999;159:1450–6.

[32] Brunelli A, Refai MA, Salati M, et al. Carbon monoxide lung diffusion capacity improves risk stratification in patients without airflow limitation: evidence for systematic measurement before lung resection. Eur J Cardiothorac Surg 2006;29:567–70.

[33] Takeda S, Funakoshi Y, Kadota Y, et al. Fall in diffusing capacity associated with induction therapy for lung cancer: a predictor of postoperative complication? Ann Thorac Surg 2006;82:232–6.

[34] Wang JS, Abboud RT, Evans KG, et al. Role of CO diffusing capacity during exercise in the preoperative evaluation for lung resection. Am J Respir Crit Care Med 2000;162:1435–44.

[35] Girish M, Trayner E Jr, Dammann O, et al. Symptom-limited stair climbing as a predictor of postoperative cardiopulmonary complications after high-risk surgery. Chest 2001;120:1147–51.

[36] Brunelli A, Al Refai M, Monteverde M, et al. Stair climbing test predicts cardiopulmonary complications after lung resection. Chest 2002;121:1106–10.

[37] Saey D, Michaud A, Couillard A, et al. Contractile fatigue, muscle morphometry, and blood lactate in chronic obstructive pulmonary disease. Am J Respir Crit Care Med 2005;171:1109–15.

[38] Washburn RA, McAuley E, Katula J, et al. The physical activity scale for the elderly (PASE) evidence for validity. J Clin Epidemiol 1999;52:643–51.

[39] Engelen MP, Schols AM, Does JD, et al. Exercise-induced lactate increase in relation to muscle substrates in patients with chronic obstructive pulmonary disease. Am J Respir Crit Care Med 2000; 162:1697–704.

[40] Dinenno FA, Seals DR, DeSouza CA, et al. Age-related decreases in basal limb blood flow in humans: time course, determinants and habitual exercise effects. J Physiol 2001;531:573–9.

[41] Coronell C, Orozco-Levi M, Mendez R, et al. Relevance of assessing quadriceps endurance in patients with COPD. Eur Respir J 2004;24:129–36.

[42] Manini TM, Everhart JE, Patel KV, et al. Daily activity energy expenditure and mortality among older adults. JAMA 2006;296:171–9.

[43] Schonhofer B, Ardes P, Geibel M, et al. Evaluation of a movement detector to measure daily activity in patients with chronic lung disease. Eur Respir J 1997;10:2814–9.

[44] Pitta F, Troosters T, Probst VS, et al. Quantifying physical activity in daily life with questionnaires and motion sensors in COPD. Eur Respir J 2006; 27:1040–55.

[45] Wechsler AS. Statistics for the rest of us. J Thorac Cardiovasc Surg 2001;122:207–8.

[46] López-Fidalgo J, Garcet-Rodriguez S, Varela G. Optimal experimental designs for prediction of morbidity after lung resection. In: Elder L, Kitsos CP, editors. Recent advances in quantitative methods in cancer and human health risk assessment. Chichester (UK): John Wiley & Sons, Ltd.; 2005. p. 345–53.

ELSEVIER
SAUNDERS

Thorac Surg Clin 18 (2008) 39–43

THORACIC
SURGERY
CLINICS

Preoperative and Postoperative Pulmonary Rehabilitation in Lung Cancer Patients

Linda Nici, MD

Pulmonary and Critical Care Section, Providence Veterans Administration Medical Center, 830 Chalkstone Avenue, Providence, RI 02908, USA

Lung cancer is the most common and deadly malignancy in the United States, with an estimated 213,380 new cases and 160,390 deaths in 2007 [1]. The average lung cancer patient has a 1-year survival, and only a fraction of patients are eligible for curative surgery.

There is a significant prevalence of chronic obstructive pulmonary disease (COPD) in patients diagnosed with lung cancer—approximately 73% in men and 53% in women [2]. Surgery in these patients can be associated with increased risk of morbidity and mortality caused by their underlying lung disease. These patients demonstrate chronic airflow obstruction and hyperinflation, resulting in increased work of breathing. They often experience difficulty mobilizing secretions and complain of dyspnea during activities of daily living, which leads to a decrease in their exercise performance. In the postoperative period, these alterations in respiratory function may lead to ineffective cough and respiratory muscle weakness or fatigue, which in turn can lead to hypoventilation with hypercapnia, hypoxemia, and respiratory failure. Therefore, this patient population is likely to have an increased incidence of significant postoperative pulmonary complications such as atelectasis, pneumonia, and acute respiratory failure requiring intubation and mechanical ventilation.

Even in those lung cancer patients who do not have underlying chronic respiratory disease, physical symptom burden, fatigue, depressive symptoms, and performance status may have a profound effect on physical function and predict poorer postoperative outcomes [3,4].

The beneficial effects of pulmonary rehabilitation (PR) in the COPD population are well-documented. This comprehensive intervention includes exercise training (both aerobic and strength training), self-management education, and nutritional and psychosocial support. It has been unequivocally shown that targeting secondary impairments associated with COPD, such as peripheral muscle, cardiac, nutritional, and psycho-social dysfunction, decreases symptoms and improves exercise capacity, functional performance, and quality of life. It is likely that PR can be of value for all patients in whom respiratory symptoms are associated with diminished functional capacity or reduced health related quality of life, including those who have non-COPD chronic respiratory disease and pulmonary malignancies [5,6].

This article begins by discussing the preoperative assessment of patients awaiting lung cancer resection, focusing mainly on those who have underlying COPD. It will then evaluate the role of PR in the preoperative and postoperative period to improve outcomes. The author will also discuss the potential role of PR to increase patient eligibility for resection.

Preoperative assessment

Common risk factors associated with postoperative complications include smoking history, advanced age, chronic cough, sputum production, severity of underlying lung disease, and obesity [7,8]. Pulmonary function tests (PFTs) are used routinely for preoperative assessment to establish the baseline severity of underlying lung disease. Although spirometry, lung volume measurements,

E-mail address: linda_nici@brown.edu

doi:10.1016/j.thorsurg.2007.10.003

and carbon monoxide diffusing capacity (DL_{CO}) are useful, multiple analyses have shown that they are poor predictors of risk, likely because of their inability to predict the patient's functional status [9]. Forced expiratory volume in 1 second (FEV_1) is not consistently reported as an independent predictor of postoperative cardiopulmonary complications, and DL_{CO} has been shown to be an independent predictor only in a minority of patients [10,11]. Despite these limitations, marginal surgical patients are generally defined as having an FEV_1 less than 1.2L, a maximum voluntary ventilation of 35% or less, a DL_{CO} of 35% or less, or hypercapnia greater than 45mm Hg [12].

Exercise testing is recommended for patients who have borderline lung function to determine who should undergo lung resection [13,14]. There are numerous studies in the literature using exercise testing as a preoperative screening tool in lung cancer patients to improve the sensitivity and specificity of predicting perioperative morbidity and mortality [15–17]. Various modes of exercise testing have been implemented, including stair climbing, timed walking tests, and incremental or submaximal cycle ergometry to measure maximal oxygen consumption [18]. In general, the ability to climb three flights of stairs, a 6-minute walk distance of greater than 700 feet, oxygen saturation greater than 92% with exercise, and a maximal oxygen consumption greater than 15 mL/kg/min are indicators of good surgical outcome.

In the preoperative period, optimal medical care for patients who have chronic respiratory disease should include smoking cessation, optimal pharmacologic therapy including bronchodilators, inhaled corticosteroids, mucolytics and oxygen therapy when indicated, and prompt treatment of exacerbations.

Pulmonary rehabilitation for surgical patients other than those who have lung cancer

PR is considered standard of care and has been shown to be an integral part of the perioperative management of patients undergoing lung volume reduction surgery (LVRS) and lung transplantation [18,19].

To derive maximal benefit, patients scheduled to undergo lung transplantation complete an extensive preoperative and postoperative PR program. In these settings, PR identifies appropriate candidates for surgical intervention, prepares patients for the physical and psychological stresses of surgery, and facilitates postoperative recovery and return to optimum functional status. In lung transplantation, PR has been shown to improve exercise capacity, knowledge and understanding, and quality of life in the preoperative period [20].

All candidates for LVRS complete comprehensive PR at least 6 to 10 weeks before surgery. PR optimizes medical management, cardiopulmonary conditioning, and nutritional status. Besides optimizing preoperative physical and emotional function, PR also serves an essential role in the selection of appropriate surgical candidates. In the National Emphysema Treatment Trial (NETT), preoperative PR was able to stratify risk for these severely compromised patients [21]. Patients who have predominantly upper-lobe emphysema and a low maximal workload after rehabilitation had lower mortality, a greater probability of improvement in exercise capacity, and a greater probability of improvement in symptoms if they underwent LVRS than if they received medical therapy alone. In contrast, patients who have predominantly non–upper-lobe emphysema and a high maximal workload after rehabilitation had higher mortality if they underwent LVRS than if they received medical therapy alone.

In extrapolating NETT results to clinical practice, subgroups identified on the basis of post-rehabilitation exercise capacity may prove to have important ramifications in other surgical situations, such as lung cancer resection. Up to 20% of patients enrolled in NETT changed their subgroup designation after rehabilitation. The majority of these patients, about two thirds, went from the low-exercise subgroup to the high-exercise subgroup. This improvement in exercise capacity might enable borderline surgical patients to undergo potentially curative surgery for lung cancer; however, there are few data to support this premise.

There are scarce data available on the use of PR in other surgical situations. A single small study evaluated the efficacy of short-term PR in COPD patients undergoing coronary artery bypass graft surgery [22]. Postoperative peak expiratory flow rates and inspiratory capacity were higher in the group that received a preoperative training package that included health education, exercise reconditioning, breathing retraining, nutritional counseling, energy conservation, and stress management. More impressively, postoperative ventilation time, postoperative complications, and hospital stay were significantly lower in the PR group than in the control group.

Pulmonary rehabilitation for patients undergoing lung resection surgery for lung cancer

The goal of management for patients undergoing lung resection is to optimize airflow, prevent and treat complications such as hypoxemia and infections, decrease symptoms, and improve functional status and quality of life. PR can provide this forum both in the preoperative and postoperative periods.

As yet, there are no robust data to recommend the routine use of preoperative PR for patients who have lung cancer. This may be caused, in part, by the relatively brief period of time between cancer diagnosis and surgery, which does not typically allow for participation in standard 8- to 12-week outpatient rehabilitation programs. A study by Bozcuk and Martin [23], however, showed that treatment delays up to 48 days appear to have no effect on survival. Because exercise capacity appears to be the best predictor of postoperative complications, it stands to reason that an intervention that can modify this parameter could significantly impact surgical outcomes. More importantly, and as discussed previously, exercise capacity may also discriminate between patients who can and cannot tolerate surgery, thereby allowing a greater number of patients to receive a potentially curative treatment option.

The National Cancer Institute is currently funding a randomized study to evaluate the effects of preoperative PR on surgical outcomes, post-lung cancer resection [24,25]. It will enroll 120 patients randomized to 4 weeks of standardized PR before surgery versus usual care. Outcomes include length of stay in hospital, duration of mechanical ventilation, duration of intensive care unit (ICU) stay, incidence of postoperative pulmonary complications, and changes in spirometry, 6-minute walk test, maximal oxygen consumption, and health status at 3 months after hospital discharge. After study completion, patients will be followed for 5 years.

Currently, there is a single pilot study looking at preoperative PR in lung cancer patients in the literature. Cesario and colleagues [26] enrolled eight lung cancer patients who, despite a favorable clinical stage, were denied surgery based on poor pulmonary function. They underwent a 4-week (20 sessions) PR program that included incremental symptom-limited aerobic exercise, breathing exercises, and educational sessions. Exercise endurance was measured by 6-minute walking test. All study patients improved their exercise capacity and were subsequently operated on with no mortality and a 25% morbidity (2/8 with postoperative hemorrhage and atrial fibrillation). These authors found that the patients who had the worst initial pulmonary function and exercise capacity received the most benefits from PR. Although these data are promising, clearly, larger controlled trials must be done before these results can be generalized.

In another related study, 32 patients who had COPD undergoing lung resection for lung cancer received either incentive spirometry and inspiratory muscle training for 2 weeks before surgery or standard care [27]. Postoperative inspiratory muscle strength, as measured by maximum inspiratory pressure, increased significantly in the treated group, but remained unchanged in the control group. No data were presented on clinical outcomes. Wilson described a 3-week pulmonary rehabilitation exercise program (PREP) at Memorial Sloan Kettering Cancer Center that included individualized home-based aerobic exercise and breathing exercises [28]. Unfortunately, there is no follow-up information on clinical outcomes.

Varela and colleagues [29] evaluated the cost-effectiveness of a respiratory physiotherapy program in patients undergoing lobectomy. The program started the day before surgery and continued through the day of discharge. It consisted of aerobic exercise on a treadmill and bicycle, coughing and breathing exercises, and shoulder and arm exercises. These authors found that the prevalence of atelectasis and mean hospital stay decreased without increasing the cost of the procedure in this group of patients as compared with historical controls.

There are two studies in the literature that evaluate the role of postoperative PR in lung cancer patients. One study examined 25 patients who accepted PR after lung resection compared with 186 who refused [30]. Respiratory function (FEV_1, forced expiratory vital capacity [FVC], peak expiratory flow [PEF]) and exercise capacity (6-minute walk distance) improved in patients undergoing PR. A reverse trend was observed in the controls, in whom many parameters decreased 1 month after surgery. In the other study, 10 patients who had severely impaired function following lung cancer treatment (9 surgical, 1 medical) were assessed before and after an 8-week inpatient PR program [31]. Despite the lack of change in pulmonary function, all patients significantly improved their exercise capacity as measured by 6-minute walk distance and peak cycling load.

There is clear rationale for the use of preoperative PR, which may impact on survival if more patients are able to undergo curative resection. Likewise, the use of postoperative PR should positively impact on functional status and quality of life in this patient population. Whether larger, randomized control trials will substantiate these hypotheses remains to be seen.

Other indications for pulmonary rehabilitation in lung cancer patients

In addition to its role in the management of surgical patient who has lung cancer, PR may also be of benefit to patients receiving chemotherapy. Aerobic exercise has been shown to be effective in reducing fatigue and psychological stress induced by systemic chemotherapy [32,33].

Summary

The benefits derived from comprehensive PR, when applied to patients who have lung cancer, should have significant impact on both survival and health status. Because PR is known to improve exercise capacity, it is reasonable to expect that this treatment modality may provide more patients with a potential cure. In addition, improvement in symptoms and quality of life can prove critically important when long-term survival is not an outcome that can be impacted on. Studies thus far support the value of this treatment modality in the global approach to patients who have lung cancer. Future well-designed clinical trials will need to corroborate these findings. We look forward to improving lung cancer outcomes with the widespread use of pulmonary rehabilitation.

References

[1] National Cancer Institute. Lung cancer. Available at: http://www.cancer.gov/cancertopics/types/lung. Accessed October 2007.

[2] Loganathan RS, Stover DE, Shi W, et al. Prevalence of COPD in women compared to men around the time of diagnosis of primary lung cancer. Chest 2006;129:1305–12.

[3] Doorenbos A, Given B, Given C, et al. Physical functioning: effect of behavioral intervention for symptoms among individuals with cancer. Nurs Res 2006;30:161–71.

[4] Hopwood P, Stephens RJ. Depression in patients with lung cancer: prevalence and risk factors derived from quality-of-life data. J Clin Oncol 2000;18: 893–903.

[5] Nici L, Donner C, Wouters E, et al. American thoracic society/European respiratory society statement on pulmonary rehabilitation. Am J Respir Crit Care Med 2006;173:1390–413.

[6] Ries AL, Bauldoff GS, Carlin BW, et al. Pulmonary rehabilitation: joint ACCP/AACVPR evidence-based clinical practice guidelines. Chest 2007;131:4S–42S.

[7] Reilly JJ, Mentzer SJ, Sugarbaker DJ. Preoperative assessment of patients undergoing pulmonary resection. Chest 1993;103:342S–5S.

[8] Wang JS. Pulmonary function tests in preoperative pulmonary evaluation. Respir Med 2004;98:598–605.

[9] Wang JS, Abboud RT, Evans KG, et al. Role of CO diffusing capacity during exercise in the preoperative evaluation for lung resection. Am J Respir Crit Care Med 2000;162(4 Pt 1):1435–44.

[10] Wang J, Olak J, Ultmann RE, et al. Assessment of pulmonary complications after lung resection. Ann Thorac Surg 1999;67(5):1444–7.

[11] Szekely LA, Oelberg DA, Wright C, et al. Preoperative predictors of operative morbidity and mortality in COPD patients undergoing lung volume reduction surgery. Chest 1997;111:550–8.

[12] Bolliger CT, Jordan P, Soler M, et al. Exercise capacity as a predictor of postoperative complications in lung resection candidates. Am J Respir Crit Care Med 1995;151:1472–80.

[13] American College of Chest Physicians. Diagnosis and management of lung cancer: ACCP evidence-based guidelines. Chest 2007;132(Suppl 3):1S–42S.

[14] British Thoracic Society. Guidelines on the selection of patients with lung cancer for surgery. Thorax 2201; 56(2):89–108.

[15] Brustsche MH, Spiliopoulos A, Bolliger CT, et al. Exercise capacity and extent of resection as predictors of surgical risk in lung cancer. Eur Respir J 2000;15(5):828–32.

[16] Villani F, Busia A. Preoperative evaluation of patients submitted to pneumonectomy for lung carcinoma: role of exercise testing. Tumori 2004;90(4):405–9.

[17] Datta D, Lahiri B. Preoperative evaluation of patients undergoing lung resection surgery. Chest 2003;123:2096–103.

[18] Palmer SM, Tapson VF. Pulmonary rehabilitation in the surgical patient. Respir Care Clin N Am 1998;4(1):71–83.

[19] Takaoka ST, Weinacker AB. The value of perioperative pulmonary rehabilitation. Thorac Surg Clin 2005;15:203–11.

[20] Manzetti JD, Hoffman LA, Sereika SM, et al. Exercise, education and quality of life in lung transplantation candidates. J Heart Lung Transplant 1994;13: 297–305.

[21] National Emphysema Treatment Trial Group. A randomized trial comparing lung volume reduction surgery with medical therapy for severe emphysema. N Engl J Med 2003;348(21):2059–73.

[22] Rajendran AJ, Pandurangi UM, Murali R, et al. Pre-operative pulmonary rehabilitation for patients of chronic obstructive pulmonary disease undergoing coronary bypass graft surgery. Indian Heart J 1998;50:531–4.
[23] Bozcuk H, Martin C. Does treatment delay affect survival in non-small cell lung cancer? A retrospective analysis for a single UK center. Lung Cancer 2001;43:243–52.
[24] Benzo R. Randomized study of pulmonary rehabilitation in patients with moderate to severe chronic obstructive pulmonary disease who require lung resection for lung cancer. National Cancer Institute clinical trial. Available at: http://www.cancer.gov/search/ViewClinicalTrials. Accessed October 2007.
[25] Benzo RP. Pulmonary rehabilitation in lung cancer. J Cardiopulm Rehabil Prev 2007;27(2):61–4.
[26] Cesario A, Ferri L, Galetta D, et al. Pre-operative pulmonary rehabilitation and surgery for lung cancer. Lung Cancer 2007;57:118–9.
[27] Weiner P, Man A, Weiner M, et al. The effect of incentive spirometry and inspiratory muscle training on pulmonary function after lung resection. J Thorac Cardiovasc Surg 1997;113:552–7.
[28] Wilson DJ. Pulmonary rehabilitation exercise program for high-risk thoracic surgical patients. Chest Surg Clin N Am 1997;7(4):697–706.
[29] Varela G, Ballesteros E, Jimenez MF, et al. Cost-effectiveness of prophylactic respiratory physiolotherapy in pulmonary lobectomy. Eur J Cardiothorac Surg 2006;29:216–20.
[30] Cesario A, Ferri L, Galetta D, et al. Post-operative respiratory rehabilitation after lung resection for non-small cell lung cancer. Lung Cancer 2007;57:175–80.
[31] Spruit MA, Janssen PP, Willemsen SC, et al. Exercise capacity before and after an 8-week multidisciplinary inpatient rehabilitation program in lung cancer patients: a pilot study. Lung Cancer 2006;52:257–60.
[32] Adamson L, Midtgaard J, Anderson C, et al. Transforming the nature of fatigue through exercise: qualitative findings from a multidimensional exercise program in cancer patients undergoing chemotherapy. Eur J Cancer Care 2004;13:362–70.
[33] Dimeo FC, Fetscher S, Lange W, et al. Effects of aerobic exercise on physical performance and incidence of treatment-related complications after high-dose chemotherapy. Blood 1997;1(90):3390–4.

ELSEVIER
SAUNDERS

Thorac Surg Clin 18 (2008) 45–59

THORACIC
SURGERY
CLINICS

Preoperative Cardiac Evaluation of Lung Resection Candidates

Steven L. Cohn, MD, FACP[a,b,*]

[a]*Division of General Internal Medicine, SUNY Downstate Medical Center, 450 Clarkson Avenue, Brooklyn, NY 11203, USA*

[b]*Medical Consultation Service, Kings County Hospital, 450 Clarkson Avenue, Box 68, Brooklyn, NY 11203, USA*

Lung cancer remains the leading cause of death from cancer in the United States (29% of all cancer deaths). In 2006 it was estimated that there were 174,000 new cases diagnosed and 162,000 deaths, with an overall 5-year survival rate of only 15% [1]. Lung resection provides the best chance for cure of this disease; the survival rate for localized disease is 50%, but only 16% of lung cancers are diagnosed at this early stage.

Patients who have lung cancer usually have significant comorbidities. The most important postoperative complications are cardiopulmonary, so the preoperative assessment should focus on these systems. The goal of preoperative evaluation is to assess the patient's risk of developing complications, optimize medical status, and recommend perioperative risk reduction strategies. Counseling and discussion with the patient and family regarding risk, surgical and nonsurgical options, expectations, and needs are imperative before making a decision as to any preoperative workup and overall treatment plan.

This article summarizes the main aspects of preoperative cardiac evaluation. (The pulmonary aspects are discussed in other articles in this issue.) Unfortunately, there is little information from clinical trials or guidelines specific to cardiac risk in the patient undergoing lung resection; therefore much of this discussion focuses on preoperative cardiac risk in general in an attempt to extrapolate these data to the lung resection candidate. The patient who has lung cancer has a potentially fatal disease, and it is important to avoid unnecessary or prolonged delays to evaluate or treat other medical comorbidities. In general these patients need to have surgery performed within a month or two of their diagnosis to minimize the chance of the disease spreading. In this respect the approach may differ significantly from that for a patient undergoing purely elective surgery.

Initial evaluation

Once the diagnosis of lung cancer has been made, initial evaluation involves a multidisciplinary team to assess the patient for curative resection. This assessment includes tests to determine the extent of disease and the patient's cardiopulmonary status.

The first step in assessing risk is a good history and physical examination. The consultant should look for any significant comorbid conditions in the medical history and ascertain their severity and stability. One should ask about tobacco use and whether the patient is still smoking. The patient's current medications need to be reviewed. This review should include prescription, over-the-counter, and herbal medications and the patient's compliance with the prescribed regimen. In the review of systems, chest pain, shortness of breath, and exercise capacity are important in assessing the patient's functional status. Important findings on the physical examination include the vital signs, use of accessory muscles, rales, rhonchi, or wheezing, heart murmurs, S3 or jugular vein distension, and leg edema.

Basic laboratory tests and diagnostic studies are directed by the patient's comorbid conditions;

* Medical Consultation Service, Kings County Hospital, 450 Clarkson Avenue, Box 68, Brooklyn, NY 11203.

E-mail address: steven.cohn@downstate.edu

1547-4127/08/$ - see front matter
doi:10.1016/j.thorsurg.2007.11.006

more detailed and specific tests of pulmonary function are performed subsequently. These latter tests include spirometry and possibly anatomic or quantitative assessment of lung function and exercise testing.

Risk factors

Risk factors can be divided into those related to the surgical procedure and those specific to the patient.

Surgical risk factors

One of the major risk factors is the extent of surgery planned, with a pneumonectomy carrying a higher risk than a lobectomy or segmental resection. Loss of functional lung tissue and the decline in pulmonary function are affected to various degrees by the different surgical procedures. Compared with the preoperative value, a rough estimate of the expected decline in postoperative predicted forced expiratory volume in 1 second (FEV_1) is a 50% reduction after a pneumonectomy, a 20% reduction after a lobectomy, and 5% per segment reduction after a segmental resection. Specific tests to evaluate preoperative and postoperative pulmonary function are discussed elsewhere.

Other surgical risk factors include the surgical approach or technique, type of anesthesia and analgesia, surgeon's experience, and hospital volume, personnel, and resources.

Patient-specific risk factors

In the history, potential risk factors for postoperative cardiovascular complications include age, known cardiac disease (coronary artery disease [CAD], heart failure, valvular disease, arrhythmias), cerebrovascular disease, hypertension, diabetes mellitus, hyperlipidemia, cigarette smoking, coexisting pulmonary disease (particularly chronic obstructive pulmonary disease [COPD]), renal insufficiency, and pretreatment with chemotherapy (which may decrease the diffusing capacity of the lungs for carbon dioxide [DLCO]).

Age

Postoperative pulmonary complication rates increase with advancing age from the mid-50s on. This increase is similar to findings for noncardiac, nonthoracic surgery noted in the American College of Physicians (ACP) guidelines for postoperative pulmonary complications [2] and occurs slightly earlier than the age usually quoted for cardiac complications ($\geq$ 70 years). Age per se probably is not the actual risk factor but is a marker for subclinical disease and decreased cardiopulmonary reserve. As noted by the American College of Chest Physician guidelines, age alone should not be used as a criterion to deny a patient potentially curative lung surgery [3].

Ischemic heart disease

The timing of a previous myocardial infarction (MI) is important because a recent MI (within the past 30 days) represents a major risk factor for perioperative cardiac complications. In the past, it was believed that elective surgery should be delayed for 6 months after an MI based on Goldman's original risk index, but the American College of Cardiology (ACC)/American Heart Association (AHA) guidelines decreased this interval to 4 to 6 weeks [4]. Before the use of routine risk stratification and early intervention with thrombolytics and now percutaneous coronary intervention (PCI), time was used as a factor in separating the higher-risk from lower-risk patients.

The medical consultant needs to assess the functional status, severity, and stability of cardiac symptoms in a patient who has CAD or heart failure. Unstable angina and New York Heart Association (NYHA) class III or IV angina are major risk factors that warrant further investigation and treatment before elective surgery. Mild, stable angina (class I–II) probably is best managed medically and usually does not warrant further cardiac testing preoperatively. Medical management of CAD is discussed later.

Heart failure

Patients who have symptoms or signs of heart failure need to be medically optimized before undergoing surgery. A history of heart failure or compensated heart failure represents less of a risk than acute heart failure.

Although the results of two-dimensional echocardiography have not predicted postoperative ischemic cardiac complications consistently, an ejection fraction of less than 35% has been associated with increased mortality, and patients who have ejection fractions of less than 20% often have been excluded from perioperative cardiac risk clinical trials. A retrospective study of 46 patients who underwent lung resection found that routinely performed multigated angiograms (MUGA) did not improve the ability to predict postoperative cardiopulmonary complications [5]. Recently, several studies have shown preoperative brain natriuretic protein (BNP) levels to correlate with postoperative cardiac complications including atrial fibrillation (AF) [6]; however, it is not clear how this marker would change perioperative management, and it is not yet routine practice to obtain these levels.

Valvular heart disease

Symptomatic severe or critical aortic stenosis has been noted in various risk indices to increase the risk of perioperative cardiac complications for noncardiac surgery and would normally be an indication for aortic valve replacement. Time may not permit valve replacement, however, or a patient may be deemed to be at too high a risk or may refuse cardiac surgery. Rarely, valvotomy may be an option, but when no intervention is planned, medical management to optimize hemodynamic status preoperatively and intraoperatively is imperative, and such patients have been able to undergo their noncardiac procedure successfully.

Mitral stenosis, especially if associated with heart failure, also is a risk factor for perioperative cardiac complications. Other valvular lesions including aortic and mitral regurgitation usually are better tolerated and usually are not associated with postoperative complications.

Arrhythmias

The patient may give a history of having an arrhythmia, or it may be noted on physical examination or ECG. The presence of atrial premature contractions, premature ventral contractions, or non-sinus rhythm may indicate underlying cardiac disease but rarely requires antiarrhythmic treatment unless it is hemodynamically significant (eg, supraventricular tachycardia, symptomatic bradycardia). Postoperative supraventricular arrhythmias (SVAs) are common (seen in 15%–30% of patients) after thoracic surgery.

Conduction defects, such as first-degree atrioventricular (AV) block, second-degree AV block Mobitz I, and bundle branch blocks are not associated with increased postoperative complications and do not require any specific treatment. Mobitz II and third-degree AV block are indications for cardiac pacing. A patient who has a pacemaker or automatic implantable cardioverter defibrillator should be evaluated preoperatively by a cardiologist with interrogation of the device and recommendations for its perioperative management.

Hypertension

Hypertension is at best a minor predictor of postoperative complications. Although there are no evidence-based guidelines correlating a specific level of blood pressure with increased risk, a systolic blood pressure above 180 mm Hg and a diastolic blood pressure above 110 mm Hg often are quoted. Hypertensive patients are more likely to experience intraoperative blood pressure lability and postoperative hypertension than are nonhypertensive patients. Antihypertensive medication and better preoperative blood pressure control may minimize some of these changes, but in general increased blood pressure rarely should be a reason to cancel surgery. The cause of the hypertension (eg, pheochromocytoma) and evidence of end-organ damage are more important than the baseline blood pressure itself in predicting complications.

Hyperlipidemia

There is no evidence linking any specific level of total cholesterol or low-density cholesterol to postoperative cardiac complications. Once again, evidence of end-organ damage probably is more predictive than cholesterol levels. Multiple observational studies suggest that perioperative use of statins may be associated with decreased complication rates, particularly in patients undergoing vascular surgery. Patients who have CAD, cerebrovascular disease, peripheral arterial disease, diabetes mellitus, and hyperlipidemia already have independent indications for statin therapy; although studies are investigating their role, there is no current recommendation to begin statins prophylactically in the absence of one of these indications.

Cigarette smoking

Although smoking is risk factor for developing cardiovascular disease, it has not been cited as a predictor of postoperative cardiac complications. Current smokers, however, are more likely to develop postoperative pulmonary complications than are nonsmokers. Evidence suggests that smokers need to quit at least 4 to 8 weeks before surgery to minimize this risk. Although several studies reported an increased risk in patients who had stopped smoking recently (< 2–4 weeks) before surgery, other studies showed no difference, and the long-term benefit of cigarette cessation should outweigh any theoretical or minor risk of stopping smoking shortly before surgery.

Chronic obstructive pulmonary disease

Postoperative pulmonary complications, especially with thoracic surgery, are more common than cardiac complications, and coexisting cardiac and pulmonary disease may place patients at increased risk for complications of both systems. COPD in general carries a twofold risk for developing postoperative pulmonary complications but rarely is mentioned as a predictor of cardiac complications. The severity of COPD, based on pulmonary function tests and symptoms, is related to postoperative complications. Medical therapy with bronchodilators, steroids, and occasionally antibiotics to optimize pulmonary status may improve outcome. Lung expansion maneuvers are also helpful.

Functional status

The patient's ability to exercise, whether measured by activities of daily living, stair climbing, shuttle walk or 6-minute-walk tests, or formal exercise testing, is an important predictor of both cardiac and pulmonary complications. The ACC guidelines use four metabolic equivalents (METS) as a cutoff for adequate exercise capacity. This roughly correlates with the ability to walk two blocks at 3 miles per hour on level ground or to climb a flight of stairs without stopping. A more extensive discussion of formal exercise capacity, including the use of maximum oxygen consumption and cardiopulmonary exercise testing, to assess pulmonary risk is discussed elsewhere.

Laboratory and diagnostic tests

Various preoperative test results have been found to be associated with or to predict postoperative cardiac or pulmonary complications.

Hematocrit. Two recent studies, one in patients who had undergone coronary artery bypass grafting (CABG) [7], and the other in patients undergoing noncardiac surgery [8], found preoperative anemia to correlate with postoperative adverse events; however, because of the studies' retrospective nature, it is unclear whether there is a cause-and-effect relationship rather than an association related to other comorbidities. Furthermore, even if anemia is related to postoperative complications, it has yet to be determined whether transfusion or other interventions will improve outcome.

Basic metabolic panel. Chronic kidney disease, as evidenced by blood urea nitrogen levels above 20 and creatinine levels above 2.0 mg/dL, was found to be a risk factor for postoperative cardiac and pulmonary complications in multiple risk indices. Diabetes requiring insulin was a risk factor in the Lee Revised Cardiac Risk Index (RCRI) [9] and the Veterans Administration Respiratory Failure Risk Index [10].

Albumin. Serum albumin levels below 3.5 g/dL was a marker for postoperative pulmonary complications; however, even hyperalimentation failed to improve outcome.

ECG

Evidence of a recent or previous MI is probably the most important ECG finding associated with postoperative cardiac complications. Hemodynamically significant arrhythmias are also risk predictors and require treatment before elective surgery.

Cardiac risk indices and algorithms

Various tools have been developed in an attempt to improve risk stratification and predict postoperative complications with the intent to intervene to reduce that risk. These tools, however, cannot totally replace a physician's judgment for an individual patient, especially because evidence is still lacking in certain areas.

Goldman's original Cardiac Risk Index was the first prospective multivariate analysis in the field [11]. It subsequently was modified by Detsky and colleagues [12], and this modification later formed the basis for the now outdated ACP guidelines [13]. These studies, however, included few thoracic surgery patients.

The most widely used risk index for predicting major postoperative cardiac complications after noncardiac surgery is the RCRI [9].

The six independent risk predictors in the index include ischemic heart disease, heart failure, cerebrovascular disease, chronic renal insufficiency (creatinine level > 2), diabetes mellitus treated with insulin, and high-risk surgery.

Patients can be classified as low (no or one risk factor), intermediate (two factors), or high (three or more factors) risk with corresponding postoperative cardiac complication rates of approximately 1%, 5%, and 10%, respectively. This index, however, did not make recommendations regarding preoperative cardiac work-up or perioperative management.

The recently updated ACC/AHA guidelines use clinical risk factors [4] (Box 1), functional capacity, and surgery-specific risk and do incorporate the RCRI concept into the algorithm.

Adequate functional capacity (moderate, good, or excellent) is defined as four or more METS and can be determined from a recent exercise test (if done) or estimated from the ability to perform activities of daily living. The Duke Activity Status Index can be used in this regard [14]. A patient who can walk at least two blocks at a rate of 3 miles per hour on level ground or climb one flight of stairs without stopping probably has an estimated exercise capacity of at least four METS.

Surgical procedures are classified as low risk (< 1% risk of cardiac complications; eg, endoscopic, ambulatory, or superficial procedures not invading a body cavity), intermediate risk (1%–5% risk of complications; eg, intraperitoneal, intrathoracic, orthopedic, head and neck, and carotid endarterectomy surgery), or high risk (> 5% risk of cardiac complications; eg, aortic and major vascular procedures, peripheral vascular surgery).

These items are incorporated into the new algorithm as shown in Fig. 1.

1. A patient requiring emergent (and the author tends to include urgent as well) surgery goes directly to the operating room (OR) without further cardiac testing. There is insufficient time for an intervention other than optimizing medical therapy.
2. Patients who have active cardiac conditions require further evaluation and treatment before undergoing elective surgery. These patients are high risk.
3. Patients scheduled for low-risk surgery can proceed to the OR without further testing because it is unlikely that any intervention will lower the already low risk of complications.
4. Patients who have good functional capacity tend to do well regardless of their other comorbid conditions (other than active cardiac conditions) and usually can proceed to surgery without further cardiac work-up.
5. Patients not meeting any of these criteria who have poor or unknown functional capacity are divided into three groups based on their clinical risk factors:
   - No clinical factors: proceed to surgery with heart rate control (beta-blockers) or consider noninvasive testing (NIT) if it will change management; in the author's opinion, patients who have clinical risk factor (if not

Box 1. American College of Cardiology/American Heart Association clinical risk factors

Active cardiac conditions

Unstable coronary syndromes
- Recent MI (within the past 30 days)
- Unstable or severe (class III/IV) angina

Decompensated heart failure (NYHA class IV, worsening, or new-onset heart failure)

Severe valvular disease (aortic stenosis with > 40 mm Hg gradient, valve area < 1 cm^2, or symptoms, or symptomatic mitral stenosis)

Significant arrhythmias (high-grade AV block, symptomatic bradyarrhythmias, ventricular arrhythmias, and SVAs)

Other clinical risk factors[a]

History of ischemic heart disease
- Old MI (> 30 days)
- Class I/II angina

History of compensated or prior heart failure

History of cerebrovascular disease

Diabetes mellitus (insulin use not specified)

Renal insufficiencySerum creatine > 2mg/dL

[a] Based on Lee Revised Cardiac Risk Index (excluding type of surgery which is incorporated elsewhere).

Data from Fleisher LA, Beckman JA, Brown KA, et al. ACC/AHA2007 Guidelines on perioperative cardiovascular evaluation and care for noncardiac surgery: executive summary: a report of the American College of Cardiology/American Heart Association Task Force on Practice Guidelines (Writing Committee to Revise the 2002 Guidelines on Perioperative Cardiovascular Evaluation for Noncardiac Surgery) developed in collaboration with the American Society of Echocardiography, American Society of Nuclear Cardiology, Heart Rhythm Society, Society of Cardiovascular Anesthesiologists, Society for Cardiovascular Angiography and Interventions, Society for Vascular Medicine and Biology, and Society for Vascular Surgery. J Am Coll Cardiol 2007;50(17):1707–32.

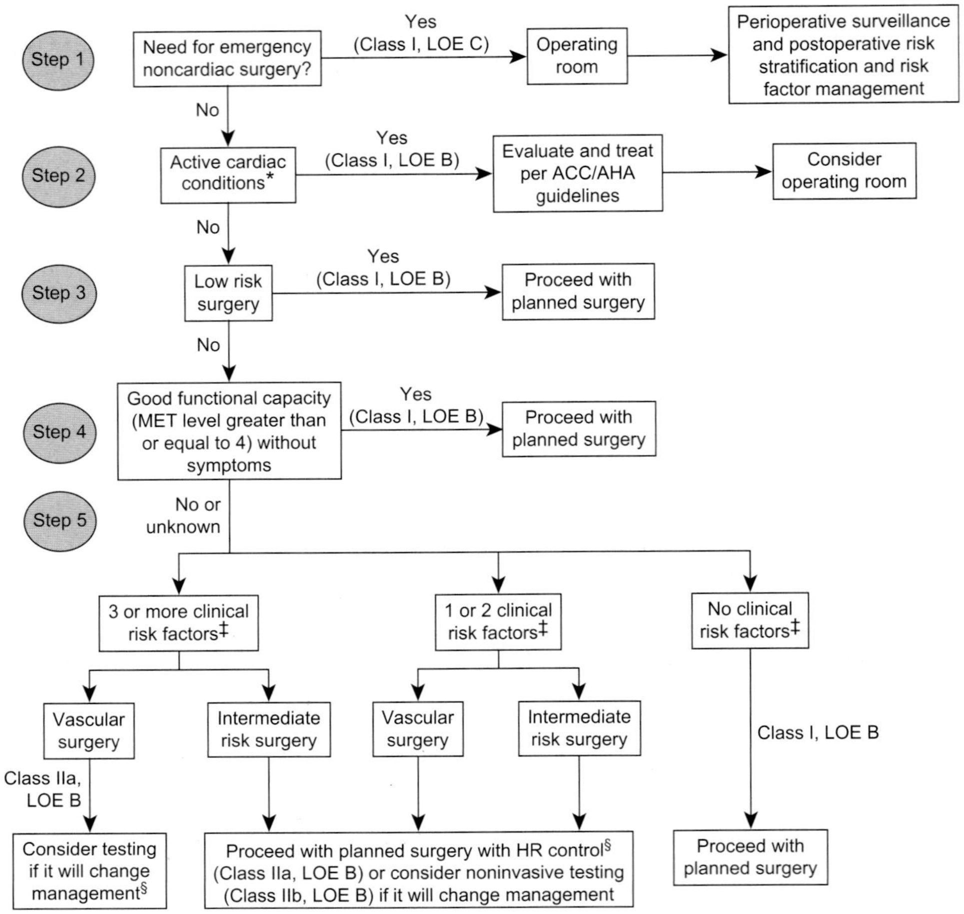

Fig. 1. Cardiac evaluation and care algorithm for noncardiac surgery based on active clinical conditions, known cardiovascular disease, or cardiac risk factors for patients 50 years of age or older. *See Box 1 for active clinical conditions. ‡, Clinical risk factors include ischemic heart disease, compensated or prior heart failure, diabetes mellitus, renal insufficiency, and cerebrovascular disease. §, Consider perioperative beta-blockade for populations in which this has been shown to reduce cardiac morbidity/mortality. ACC/AHA, American College of Cardiology/American Heart Association; HR, heart rate; LOE, level of evidence; MET, metabolic equivalent. (*Adapted from* Fleisher LA, Beckman JA, Brown KA, et al. ACC/AHA 2007 guidelines on perioperative cardiovascular evaluation and care for noncardiac surgery: executive summary: a report of the American College of Cardiology/American Heart Association Task Force on Practice Guidelines [Writing Committee to Revise the 2002 Guidelines on Perioperative Cardiovascular Evaluation for Noncardiac Surgery] developed in collaboration with the American Society of Echocardiography, American Society of Nuclear Cardiology, Heart Rhythm Society, Society of Cardiovascular Anesthesiologists, Society for Cardiovascular Angiography and Interventions, Society for Vascular Medicine and Biology, and Society for Vascular Surgery. J Am Coll Cardiol 2007;50(17):1716; with permission. Copyright © 2007, by the American College of Cardiology Foundation and the American Heart Association, Inc.)

CAD) probably belong in this category as well, based on the low risk of complications noted in the Lee study.

- Three or more clinical factors: consider testing for patients undergoing vascular surgery if it will change management; otherwise use heart rate control for vascular and nonvascular surgery.
- One or two clinical factors: proceed to surgery with heart rate control or possibly consider NIT if it will change management.

These recommendations are somewhat ambiguous because of the level of evidence, or lack thereof. Patients undergoing vascular surgery are the most widely studied group, based on their higher risk of complications, and there is more evidence to support the use of cardiac testing in this group than in intermediate-risk patients or those undergoing nonvascular surgery. This algorithm gives the consultant some leeway in deciding whether to do further cardiac tests, depending on the situation. The underlying theme of the ACC guidelines is that no test should be done unless the result will change management, but the ultimate deciding factor is whether the change in management will improve outcome.

For patients undergoing lung resection, the surgery is never emergent, but it does need to be performed in a relatively short time frame (ie, it cannot be delayed for 3 to 6 months or more). Although it is not vascular surgery, lung resection is considered to be at the high end of the intermediate-risk procedures. Many of these patients have poor exercise capacity based on their smoking history, which may cause cardiac or pulmonary disease, and it may be difficult to separate the cardiac from the pulmonary component. All patients undergoing lung resection will undergo spirometry, but only a limited number will have formal exercise testing for cardiopulmonary function.

For patients undergoing exercise ECG testing, the peak heart rate, systolic blood pressure, and rate pressure product are important as well as whether the patient achieved 85% of the target heart rate. The ischemic threshold is useful for perioperative anesthetic management. For patients unable to exercise and undergoing pharmacologic stress testing (dobutamine stress echocardiography [DSE] or dipyridamole or adenosine nuclear imaging), the number and extent of abnormalities tend to correlate with postoperative complications (new or worsening wall motion abnormalities for DSE and reperfusion defects with nuclear imaging). Although fairly comparable, DSE usually has a slightly lower rate of false positives than dipyridamole thallium imaging. The negative predictive value of these tests is high (90%–100%), but the positive predictive value is poor (15%–20%). Because adenosine and dipyridamole can cause bronchospasm, dobutamine usually is the preferred pharmacologic stressor in patients who have obstructive lung disease. Pharmacologic stress (dipyridamole thallium) is preferred for patients who have left bundle branch block because of false-positive septal perfusion defects (unrelated to CAD) with exercise myocardial perfusion imaging. Patients who have evidence of significant ischemia on NIT usually undergo coronary angiography; those who have left main or triple-vessel disease are potential candidates for CABG, whereas those who have single- or double-vessel disease may undergo PCI with or without stenting or be managed medically.

Epstein and colleagues [15] proposed a combined Cardiopulmonary Risk Index (CPRI) using Goldman's original cardiac risk index plus a pulmonary risk index (including obesity, cigarette smoking, productive cough, wheezing or rhonchi, a FEV_1/forced vital capacity < 70%, and $Paco_2$ > 45 mm Hg). When tested on 42 patients who had cardiopulmonary exercise testing before lung resection, higher CPRI scores were associated with increased incidence of postoperative complications, with a score of 4 or more having the best predictive value. In this study a CPRI score of 4 performed even better than peak oxygen consumption per unit of time. The same authors, in another study of 74 patients undergoing lung resection, found the CPRI score and the inability to exercise were independently associated with an increased risk for postoperative cardiopulmonary complications [16]. A subsequent study of 180 patients undergoing thoracic surgery reported that CPRI in general did not predict complications or death, but a score of 4 or higher was a moderate predictor of outcome for patients undergoing pneumonectomy [17]. In all three of these studies, the majority of the cardiac complications were arrhythmias or heart failure with very few MIs.

Several other scoring systems have been used to predict overall postoperative complications including cardiac and pulmonary complications.

The Charlson Comorbidity Index comprising multiple conditions was found to predict postoperative complications after surgery for non-small cell lung cancer. Grades 3 to 4 and above were the best predictors of adverse short term outcome [18]; an increasing score also predicted impaired long-term survival [19]. Other predictors of poor long-term outcome included increased age, more extensive surgery, and pathologic stage.

The Physiologic and Operative Severity Score for the Enumeration of Mortality and Morbidity (POSSUM) was predictive of postoperative complications in 250 patients undergoing lung resection surgery [20].

A scoring system using FEV percent, age, and DLCO percent (EVAD), developed from 400 patients undergoing lung resection between 1980 and 1995, was evaluated against POSSUM and CPRI in 218 patients undergoing lung resection between 1996 and 2001 [21]. Although the area under the curve was only 0.65 for overall complications with EVAD, it demonstrated a better ability to quantitate relative risk than the other two systems. None of the systems, however, predicted incremental risk for cardiac complications.

Using a different algorithm, Cagirici and colleagues [22] evaluated 128 patients undergoing pulmonary resection. Risk factors were defined as cigarette smoking, hypertension, hyperlipidemia, advanced age, diabetes mellitus, and a history of cardiac disease or angina. A patient who had two of the first three risk factors or one of the latter three factors underwent stress testing and, if stress testing was positive, coronary angiography. Only four patients were deemed to be high risk with ischemia on the stress test and CAD on angiography. Surgery was postponed in one patient, and the other three underwent CABG before lung resection, but the outcomes were not reported. Four of 95 patients classified as low risk (no risk factors and a negative stress test) and 8 of 29 patients classified as intermediate risk (cardiac disease or risk factors with a negative stress test or negative angiogram after a positive stress test) developed postoperative SVAs, but there were no MIs or deaths.

Several other studies used multivariate analyses to identify risk factors for cardiopulmonary complications after lung resection. Yano and colleagues [23] evaluated 291 patients and found that age over 70 years, pneumonectomy or combined resection, DLCO below 70%, and preoperative ECG abnormalities to be predictors of postoperative morbidity. The cardiac complications were primarily arrhythmias (8.9%; n = 26) with heart failure and MI occurring in only thee and two patients, respectively. Licker and colleagues [24] reported an operative mortality rate of 3.2% in 634 patients. Half of these deaths were attributable to cardiovascular complications, and an additional five patients had nonfatal MIs. Independent predictors for operative death included pneumonectomy, CAD, and American Society of Anesthesiologist's classification of III or IV.

Risk-reduction strategies

Prevention of myocardial ischemia/infarction

The literature is sparse regarding studies of ischemic complications in lung resection surgery. An older study reported an incidence of transient perioperative ischemia of 3.8% in 598 lung resection patients [25]. Despite mortality rates of 2% to 21%, perioperative MI occurs infrequently in patients who have no cardiac history (< 1%) but somewhat more often in patients who have had a prior MI (3%–17%). Patients who have troponin elevation after lung resection, with or without symptoms of MI, were found to be at high risk of early mortality (the acceleration factor for death after adjusting for tumor stage was 9.1) [26]. The ACC/AHA guidelines and algorithm were reviewed earlier. The question is whether, once the high-risk patient has been identified, coronary revascularization or medical therapy reduces complications.

Coronary revascularization: coronary artery bypass grafting

Observational data from patients in the Coronary Artery Surgery Study (CASS) who subsequently underwent noncardiac surgery suggested that those treated with CABG had lower rates of postoperative nonfatal MI and death than those treated medically [27]. This apparent benefit was seen only in higher-risk surgical procedures and seemed to be protective for 4 to 6 years; however, this report did not take into account the risks associated with the CABG itself—MI, stroke, and death.

The only randomized, controlled trial of coronary artery revascularization prophylaxis (CARP) versus medical therapy for noncardiac surgery failed to demonstrate a benefit in 510 patients who had stable cardiac disease undergoing elective vascular surgery [28]. Short-term (30-day) event rates were similar, approximately 3% mortality and 8% to 12% MI, and the primary outcome of long-term mortality was 23% in both groups. Of note is that both groups received intensive medical therapy with beta-blockers and statins, and patients who had more severe disease (left main coronary artery disease, left ventricular ejection fraction < 20%, and significant aortic stenosis) were excluded from the trial. In a substudy of CARP it seemed that CABG might be more protective than PCI [29]; however, in the Bypass Angioplasty Revascularization Investigation trial patients who subsequently had noncardiac surgery seemed to have lower rates of morbidity and mortality (2.5%) that were comparable for CABG and PCI patient groups [30].

Ciriaco and colleagues [31] reported results of 50 patients who had CAD undergoing lung resection. Nineteen underwent prophylactic coronary revascularization—6 CABG and 13 PCI (6 with stents)—followed by lung surgery an average of 32 days later with no mortalities. Of the 31 patients not revascularized, 15 had false-positive stress tests. Postoperative arrhythmias occurred in 21% of both groups, and there were no MIs or heart failure complications.

In the CARP trial the mean duration from randomization to vascular surgery was approximately 7 weeks. This delay may be unacceptable for patients who have lung cancer, in which case lung resection simultaneously with or shortly following CABG may be an option. For staged procedures, it is recommended that pulmonary surgery be performed 4 to 6 weeks after CABG, 1 to 2 weeks after angioplasty, and 4 to 6 weeks after bare metal stenting. Potential problems of a combined approach include risk of hemorrhage from heparin used during CABG, immunosuppressant effects of bypass leading to postoperative infections, and limited anatomic exposure depending on the surgical approach. Observational studies (Table 1) of staged or simultaneous procedures reported reasonably good cardiac outcomes, but the numbers of patients in these groups were small, and this approach probably is indicated only for a very small minority of patients who have lung cancer.

Coronary revascularization: percutaneous coronary intervention

Early reports of patients undergoing balloon angioplasty before noncardiac surgery suggested that it was associated with lower rates of perioperative cardiac complications than seen in

Table 1
Coronary revascularization and lung resection surgery

Author	Year	# Patients	Cardiac procedure	Sequence	Death/ myocardial infarction	% Mortality
Ulicny et al [57]	1992	19		S 16 L-H 3	1/0	5.2
Rosalion et al [58]	1993	10		S 10	0	0
Yokoyama et al [59]	1993	11	On pump 11	S 11	0	0
Terzi et al [60]	1994	10		L-H 8 S 2	1	10
Thomas et al [61]	1994	(21) 7	CABG 3 PCI 4 Med 12 No surg 2	H-L 7	1/1	14.3
Miller et al [62]	1994	30 15		S 30 H-L 15	2/1 0/0	4.4
Johnson et al [63]	1996	20		S 18 H-L 1 L-H 1	0	0
Rao et al [64]	1996	30		S 30	2/0	6.7
Voets et al [65]	1997	34	On pump 13 Off pump 11	S 24 H-L 9 L-H 1	5/1 1/0 0/0	17.6
Danton et al [66]	1998	13	On pump 11 Off pump 2	L-H 12 H-L 1	0	0
Mariani et al [67]	2001	3	Off pump 3	S 3	0/0	0
Ciriaco et al [31]	2002	(50) 19	CABG 6 PCI 13 Med 31	H-L 19	2	10.5
Ambrogi et al [68]	2003	14	On pump 8 Off pump 4 PCI 2	H-L 9 L-H 5	2/1 2/1	28.6
Dyszkiewicz et al [69]	2004	13	Off pump 13	H-L 13	0	0
Schoenmakers et al [70]	2007	43	On pump 28 Off pump 15	L-H 28 H-L 15	2/0 1/0	7
Totals		291		S 144 H-L 89 L-H 58	10/2 8/2 4/1	7.6

Abbreviations: H, heart; L, lung; S, simultaneous.

historical controls. As stents became the standard of care, Kaluza [32] reported poor outcomes in patients undergoing noncardiac surgery shortly after receiving a bare metal stent. A significant number of patients sustained fatal or nonfatal MIs or had major bleeding (depending on whether antiplatelet drugs were continued), but almost all postoperative complications occurred in patients who underwent stenting less than 2 weeks before surgery. Subsequent observational studies reported similar findings extending out to 6 weeks after stenting, and the recommendation was to postpone noncardiac surgery for at least 4 and preferably 6 weeks after placement of a bare metal stent [33].

A study of 32 patients undergoing lung resection within 3 months of coronary stenting (with non–drug-eluting stents) using heparin with or without aspirin reported in-stent thrombosis in three patients (9%) with one fatal outcome [34]. Two of these three thromboses occurred in patients who had received 4 weeks of dual antiplatelet therapy, so this duration of therapy may be insufficient as well. Another case report included a man undergoing lung resection 6 weeks after bare metal stenting who stopped antiplatelet therapy 2 weeks before surgery and had a fatal MI caused by stent thrombosis [35].

More recently drug-eluting stents have replaced bare metal stents, and although the long-term risk of restenosis has improved, multiple cases of late stent thrombosis have been reported. The original recommendations to continue antiplatelet therapy for 2 to 3 months after sirolimus stents and 6 months after paclitaxel stents subsequently were thought to be inadequate. The current recommendation by the ACC/AHA is to continue uninterrupted dual antiplatelet therapy with aspirin and clopidogrel for at least 12 months and, if possible, to postpone elective surgery to complete this course of antiplatelet therapy [36]. If the plan is to do lung resection surgery within a 2-month time frame, a drug-eluting stent should not be inserted. If possible, aspirin should be continued perioperatively in patients undergoing PCI, but clopidogrel usually is stopped at least 5 days before surgery. Further studies are necessary to determine optimal perioperative management of antiplatelet therapy.

Medical therapy: beta-blockers

Early studies with prophylactic beta-blockers demonstrated beneficial effects, prompting the recommendation in the 1997 ACP guidelines that this therapy be considered for patients at risk. Despite various studies, it still is unclear which patients undergoing which surgery will benefit. Atenolol, started immediately preoperatively and continued for a maximum of 7 days, resulted in decreased cardiac mortality 2 years after noncardiac surgery [37]. It also reduced the incidence of perioperative ischemia but had no effect on perioperative MI or in-hospital cardiac death. Bisoprolol, begun at least 7 days preoperatively and continued for 30 days postoperatively, significantly reduced short-term MI and death rates from 33% to 3.4% in patients undergoing vascular surgery and also improved long-term MI and mortality in patients who continued the bisoprolol [38]. Both these studies involved titrating the dose of beta-blocker to achieve heart rates between 55 and 70 beats per minute. Analysis of a large administrative database showed that beta-blocker use within 48 hours after surgery decreased hospital mortality in high-risk (RCRI $\geq$ 3) but not low-risk (RCRI 0–1) patients [39]. As noted in the ACC algorithm and CASS results, it is difficult to improve on the already low risk of complications in patients undergoing low-risk surgical procedures.

Three subsequent studies failed to demonstrate a beneficial effect of beta-blockers. The Metoprolol After Vascular Surgery [40] and Perioperative Beta-Blockade (POBBLE) [41] studies using metoprolol in patients undergoing vascular surgery had similar 30-day cardiovascular event rates in both groups, and the Diabetic Postoperative Mortality and Morbidity (DIPOM) study of diabetic patients undergoing noncardiac surgery showed no difference in the in-hospital cardiovascular event rates between groups [42]. In these studies, the beta-blocker dose was not titrated, the mean heart rates were somewhat higher than in the earlier studies, or the patients represented a heterogeneous group without documented CAD. Another observational study suggested that longer-acting beta-blockers might be better than shorter-acting ones [43].

The importance of heart rate control was demonstrated in a study by Feringa and colleagues [44], who found that beta-blocker dose and mean heart rate had a direct correlation with postoperative complications (troponin release and ischemia). Complication rates decreased as mean heart rate decreased to below 70 beats per minute. A subsequent study validated this finding by showing that tight heart rate control could obviate the need for NIT in intermediate-risk patients scheduled for vascular surgery [45]. There was no difference in complications based on whether a patient had a cardiac test performed, and the outcomes were better, regardless of test status, for patients who had heart rates of 65 beats per minute or less.

The ACC guideline recommendations [4] state that beta-blockers

- Should be continued in any patient already taking them (I(C))
- Should be given to high-risk patients undergoing vascular surgery who have evidence of ischemia on a stress test (I(B))
- Are probably recommended for patients who have CAD or high cardiac risk undergoing intermediate- to high-risk surgery (including vascular surgery (IIa(B))
- May be considered (usefulness is uncertain) in patients undergoing vascular surgery who have no clinical risk factors or patients at intermediate cardiac risk scheduled for intermediate- to high-risk surgery (IIb(C))
- Should not be given to any patient who has absolute contraindications to beta-blockers (III(C))

It is hoped that the large randomized, controlled Perioperative Ischemic Evaluation (POISE) trial of beta-blockers in more than 6000 patients undergoing various operations that now is nearing completion will help elucidate which patient groups will benefit from beta-blockers [46].

Medical therapy: alpha-agonists

It is likely that a number of patients undergoing lung resection will not be candidates for beta-blocker therapy because of their underlying pulmonary disease. A meta-analysis demonstrated a beneficial effect of alpha-agonists in the perioperative setting; however, these results were driven mainly by a drug (mivazerol) that is not available in the United States, and the benefit was restricted to patients undergoing vascular surgery [47]. A small study using clonidine (oral and transdermal) did show lower rates of perioperative ischemia and mortality but no difference in perioperative MI or other cardiac complications [48]. Despite limited data, this treatment may be an option in high-risk patients who have contraindications to beta-blockers.

Medical therapy: statins

Numerous observational studies and meta-analyses have demonstrated that perioperative statin use is associated with improved outcome after cardiac and noncardiac surgery [49]; however, only one small randomized, controlled trial showed a benefit of a composite cardiac outcome [50]. Most likely this beneficial effect results from the pleiotropic effects of statins and plaque stabilization rather than a specific effect on cholesterol levels. These pleiotropic effects include increased expression of endothelial nitric oxide synthase, generation of reductive oxygen species, reduction of endothelin-1 production, improved thrombogenic profile, and, probably the most important factor, a reduction in inflammation with reduced expression of cytokines, chemokines, adhesion molecules, and lower C-reactive protein levels. Statins may also affect heart rate variability, which has been associated with risk for MI.

There are a number of unknowns regarding the use of perioperative statins—the relationship to baseline lipid values, the optimal dose, timing, and duration of therapy, and whether the observed benefit is a class effect or if individual statins differ from each other. A recent study noted improved outcomes in patients undergoing vascular surgery receiving higher statin doses even after adjustment for the cholesterol level [51]. Despite the current pharmaceutical manufacturers' package labeling stating that statins should be discontinued before surgery, the ACC guidelines and most clinicians recommend continuing them perioperatively [52]. A safety study of perioperative statins did not reveal any increase in rhabdomyolysis or liver failure [53]. The Dutch Echocardiographic Cardiac Risk Evaluation Applying Stress ECHO trial currently is investigating whether prophylactic statins are beneficial, but at this time there is not enough evidence to make that recommendation [54].

Antiarrhythmics

Arrhythmias are the most common cardiac complications after thoracic surgery with a reported incidence usually in the range of 15% to 30%, depending on type of surgery. SVAs, mainly AF, are much more common than ventricular arrhythmias. Potential risk factors noted in various studies include older age, pre-existing cardiac disease, a preoperative heart rate higher than 72 beats per minute, N-terminal pro-B-type natriuretic peptide levels, COPD or limited pulmonary reserve, postural changes, more extensive surgical procedures, various anesthetic agents, major bleeding, or prior intrathoracic irradiation. Onset is most common 2 to 3 days postoperatively, and various drugs have been used prophylactically or for treatment once the arrhythmia occurs. Digoxin, diltiazem, and amiodarone were effective in treating postoperative SVA, but digoxin was less effective in patients who had COPD. Despite their frequent occurrence, these arrhythmias do not seem to increase perioperative mortality.

Reviews of prophylactic antiarrhythmic therapy [55,56] found

- Digoxin did not decrease the incidence of postoperative AF compared with placebo in several studies of thoracic and pulmonary surgery patients.
- Flecainide was effective in preventing or reducing arrhythmias compared with placebo or digoxin, and it also was useful in converting digoxin failures.
- Beta-blockers also were successful in reducing the incidence of postoperative AF after lung resection surgery.
- Intravenous amiodarone to prevent SVA in pulmonary surgery patients was associated with an increased incidence of acute respiratory distress syndrome (ARDS), but prophylactic oral amiodarone at a lower dose decreased the incidence of postoperative AF.
- Verapamil seemed to decrease the incidence of postoperative AF compared with placebo but was associated with hypotension and bradycardia.
- Diltiazem decreased postoperative AF after lung resection surgery, but in another study of thoracic surgery patients it was associated with hypotension.
- Magnesium sulfate significantly reduced the incidence of atrial tachyarrhythmias after noncardiac thoracic surgery in one study.
- Thoracic epidural bupivacaine was more effective than morphine in reducing supraventricular tachyarrhythmias after lung resection surgery.
- Statin use was associated with a decrease in AF after thoracic surgery independent of C-reactive protein levels.
- Corticosteroids were associated with a decreased incidence of postoperative AF after cardiothoracic surgery.

The best approach to preventing SVA after thoracic surgery remains unclear.

Heart failure/pulmonary edema

Acute heart failure requires treatment and stabilization before surgery. Optimization may include therapy with loop diuretics, angiotensin-converting enzyme inhibitors or angiotensin receptor blockers, vasodilators (hydralazine and nitrates), and in severe cases of left ventricular systolic dysfunction, inotropic agents (digoxin, dobutamine infusion) and spironolactone. Beta-blockers are not used for acute episodes of heart failure but usually are part of chronic therapy. Patients who have more severe disease (NYHA class III–IV or marked left ventricular dysfunction detected on echocardiography or MUGA) are at increased risk of developing postoperative heart failure. Impaired right heart function, acute MI, pre-existing valvular disease, and cardiac herniation are other causes of postoperative left ventricular dysfunction. Postoperative right ventricular dysfunction secondary to alterations in contractile performance and changes in right ventricular afterload may be seen within 48 hours after surgery. There is no test to predict right heart failure.

Pulmonary edema after lung resection is uncommon (incidence, 2%–4%) and is most likely to occur after pneumonectomy. It usually is noncardiac in origin, being related to an increased filtration gradient and hyperpermeability. Positive fluid balance, impaired lymphatic drainage, and surgical manipulation may be contributing factors. Treatment includes diuretics, fluid restriction, adequate oxygenation, and possibly inhaled nitric oxide. Unfortunately, mortality is high.

Summary

Patients who have lung cancer typically have both pulmonary and cardiac disease as a result of cigarette smoking and are potentially at increased risk for perioperative cardiopulmonary complications. Knowledge of risk factors and a careful preoperative assessment will help the medical team stratify the patient's level of risk and employ measures to minimize surgical risk. The available literature specific to cardiac risk and lung cancer surgery is minimal, but the general principles of preoperative cardiac risk evaluation and perioperative management have been reviewed. When considering cardiac testing and interventions, the medical consultant must remember that surgery is the treatment of choice for non-small cell lung cancer and must avoid any excessive delay that might compromise the patient's chance of a surgical cure.

References

[1] American Cancer Society Statistics. Available at: http://www.cancer.org/downloads/STT/CAFF2006PWSecured.pdf. Accessed November 5, 2007.

[2] Qaseem A, Snow V, Fitterman N, et al. Risk assessment for and strategies to reduce perioperative pulmonary complications for patients undergoing noncardiothoracic surgery: a guideline from the American College of Physicians. Ann Intern Med 2006;144(8):575–80.

[3] Colice GL, Shafazand S, Griffin JP, et al. Physiologic evaluation of the patient with lung cancer being considered for resectional surgery: ACCP evidenced-based clinical practice guidelines (2nd edition). Chest 2007;132(Suppl 3):161S–77S.

[4] Fleisher LA, Beckman JA, Brown KA, et al. ACC/AHA 2007 Guidelines on perioperative cardiovascular evaluation and care for noncardiac surgery: executive summary: a report of the American College of Cardiology/American Heart Association Task Force on Practice Guidelines (Writing Committee to Revise the 2002 Guidelines on Perioperative Cardiovascular Evaluation for Noncardiac Surgery) developed in collaboration with the American Society of Echocardiography, American Society of Nuclear Cardiology, Heart Rhythm Society, Society of Cardiovascular Anesthesiologists, Society for Cardiovascular Angiography and Interventions, Society for Vascular Medicine and Biology, and Society for Vascular Surgery. J Am Coll Cardiol 2007;50(17):1707–32.

[5] Ghent WS, Olsen GN, Hornung CA, et al. Routinely performed multigated blood pool imaging (MUGA) as a predictor of postoperative complications of lung resection. A two-year retrospective. Chest 1994;105(5):1454–7.

[6] Cardinale D, Colombo A, Sandri MT, et al. Increased perioperative N-terminal pro-B-type natriuretic peptide levels predict atrial fibrillation after thoracic surgery for lung cancer. Circulation 2007;115(11):1339–44.

[7] Kulier A, Levin J, Moser R, et al. Impact of preoperative anemia on outcome in patients undergoing coronary artery bypass graft surgery. Circulation 2007;116(5):471–9.

[8] Wu WC, Schifftner TL, Henderson WG, et al. Preoperative hematocrit levels and postoperative outcomes in older patients undergoing noncardiac surgery. JAMA 2007;297(22):2481–8.

[9] Lee TH, Marcantonio ER, Mangione CM, et al. Derivation and prospective validation of a simple index for prediction of cardiac risk of major noncardiac surgery. Circulation 1999;100(10):1043–9.

[10] Arozullah AM, Daley J, Henderson WG, et al. Multifactorial risk index for predicting postoperative respiratory failure in men after major noncardiac surgery. The National Veterans Administration Surgical Quality Improvement Program. Ann Surg 2000;232(2):242–53.

[11] Goldman L, Caldera DL, Nussbaum SR, et al. Multifactorial index of cardiac risk in noncardiac surgical procedures. N Engl J Med 1977;297(16):845–50.

[12] Detsky AS, Abrams HB, Forbath N, et al. Cardiac assessment for patients undergoing noncardiac surgery. A multifactorial clinical risk index. Arch Intern Med 1986;146(11):2131–4.

[13] Palda VA, Detsky AS. Perioperative assessment and management of risk from coronary artery disease. Ann Intern Med 1997;127(4):313–28.

[14] Hlatky MA, Boineau RE, Higginbotham MB, et al. A brief self-administered questionnaire to determine functional capacity (the Duke Activity Status Index). Am J Cardiol 1989;64(10):651–4.

[15] Epstein SK, Faling LJ, Daly BD, et al. Predicting complications after pulmonary resection. Preoperative exercise testing vs a multifactorial cardiopulmonary risk index. Chest 1993;104(3):694–700.

[16] Epstein SK, Faling LJ, Daly BD, et al. Inability to perform bicycle ergometry predicts increased morbidity and mortality after lung resection. Chest 1995;107(2):311–6.

[17] Melendez JA, Carlon VA. Cardiopulmonary risk index does not predict complications after thoracic surgery. Chest 1998;114(1):69–75.

[18] Birim O, Maat AP, Kappetein AP, et al. Validation of the Charlson Comorbidity Index in patients with operated primary non-small cell lung cancer. Eur J Cardiothorac Surg 2003;23(1):30–4.

[19] Birim O, Kappetein AP, Bogers AJ. Charlson Comorbidity Index as a predictor of long-term outcome after surgery for nonsmall cell lung cancer. Eur J Cardiothorac Surg 2005;28(5):759–62.

[20] Brunelli A, Fianchini A, Xiume F, et al. Evaluation of the POSSUM scoring system in lung surgery. Physiological and operative severity score for the enumeration of mortality and morbidity. Thorac Cardiovasc Surg 1998;46(3):141–6.

[21] Ferguson MK, Durkin AE. A comparison of three scoring systems for predicting complications after major lung resection. Eur J Cardiothorac Surg 2003;23(1):35–42.

[22] Cagirici U, Nalbantgil S, Cakan A, et al. A new algorithm for preoperative cardiac assessment in patients undergoing pulmonary resection. Tex Heart Inst J 2005;32(2):159–62.

[23] Yano T, Yokoyama H, Fukuyama Y, et al. The current status of postoperative complications and risk factors after a pulmonary resection for primary lung cancer. A multivariate analysis. Eur J Cardiothorac Surg 1997;11(3):445–9.

[24] Licker M, de Perrot M, Hohn L, et al. Perioperative mortality and major cardio-pulmonary complications after lung surgery for non-small cell carcinoma. Eur J Cardiothorac Surg 1999;15(3):314–9.

[25] von Knorring J, Lepantalo M, Lindgren L, et al. Cardiac arrhythmias and myocardial ischemia after thoracotomy for lung cancer. Ann Thorac Surg 1992;53(4):642–7.

[26] Lim E, Li Choy L, Flaks L, et al. Detected troponin elevation is associated with high early mortality after

lung resection for cancer. J Cardiothorac Surg 2006; 1:37–45.

[27] Eagle KA, Rihal CS, Mickel MC, et al. Cardiac risk of noncardiac surgery: influence of coronary disease and type of surgery in 3368 operations. CASS Investigators and University of Michigan Heart Care Program. Coronary Artery Surgery Study. Circulation 1997;96(6):1882–7.

[28] McFalls EO, Ward HB, Moritz TE, et al. Coronary-artery revascularization before elective major vascular surgery. N Engl J Med 2004; 351(27):2795–804.

[29] Ward HB, Kelly RF, Thottapurathu L, et al. Coronary artery bypass grafting is superior to percutaneous coronary intervention in prevention of perioperative myocardial infarctions during subsequent vascular surgery. Ann Thorac Surg 2006; 82(3):795–800 [discussion: 800–1].

[30] Hassan SA, Hlatky MA, Boothroyd DB, et al. Outcomes of noncardiac surgery after coronary bypass surgery or coronary angioplasty in the Bypass Angioplasty Revascularization Investigation (BARI). Am J Med 2001;110(4):260–6.

[31] Ciriaco P, Carretta A, Calori G, et al. Lung resection for cancer in patients with coronary arterial disease: analysis of short-term results. Eur J Cardiothorac Surg 2002;22(1):35–40.

[32] Kaluza GL, Joseph J, Lee JR, et al. Catastrophic outcomes of noncardiac surgery soon after coronary stenting. J Am Coll Cardiol 2000;35(5):1288–94.

[33] Wilson SH, Fasseas P, Orford JL, et al. Clinical outcome of patients undergoing non-cardiac surgery in the two months following coronary stenting. J Am Coll Cardiol 2003;42(2):234–40.

[34] Brichon PY, Boitet P, Dujon A, et al. Perioperative in-stent thrombosis after lung resection performed within 3 months of coronary stenting. Eur J Cardiothorac Surg 2006;30(5):793–6.

[35] Marcucci C, Chassot PG, Gardaz JP, et al. Fatal myocardial infarction after lung resection in a patient with prophylactic preoperative coronary stenting. Br J Anaesth 2004;92(5):743–7.

[36] Grines CL, Bonow RO, Casey DE Jr, et al. Prevention of premature discontinuation of dual antiplatelet therapy in patients with coronary artery stents: a science advisory from the American Heart Association, American College of Cardiology, Society for Cardiovascular Angiography and Interventions, American College of Surgeons, and American Dental Association, with representation from the American College of Physicians. Circulation 2007; 115(6):813–8.

[37] Mangano DT, Layug EL, Wallace A, et al. Effect of atenolol on mortality and cardiovascular morbidity after noncardiac surgery. Multicenter Study of Perioperative Ischemia Research Group. N Engl J Med 1996;335(23):1713–20.

[38] Poldermans D, Boersma E, Bax JJ, et al. The effect of bisoprolol on perioperative mortality and myocardial infarction in high-risk patients undergoing vascular surgery. Dutch Echocardiographic Cardiac Risk Evaluation Applying Stress Echocardiography Study Group. N Engl J Med 1999; 341(24):1789–94.

[39] Lindenauer PK, Pekow P, Wang K, et al. Perioperative beta-blocker therapy and mortality after major noncardiac surgery. N Engl J Med 2005;353(4):349–61.

[40] Yang H, Raymer K, Butler R, et al. The effects of perioperative beta-blockade: results of the metoprolol after vascular surgery (MaVS) study, a randomized controlled trial. Am Heart J 2006; 152(5):983–90.

[41] Brady AR, Gibbs JS, Greenhalgh RM, et al. Perioperative beta-blockade (POBBLE) for patients undergoing infrarenal vascular surgery: results of a randomized double-blind controlled trial. J Vasc Surg 2005;41(4):602–9.

[42] Juul AB, Wetterslev J, Gluud C, et al. Effect of perioperative beta blockade in patients with diabetes undergoing major non-cardiac surgery: randomised placebo controlled, blinded multicentre trial. BMJ 2006;332(7556):1482–8.

[43] Redelmeier D, Scales D, Kopp A. Beta blockers for elective surgery in elderly patients: population based, retrospective cohort study. BMJ 2005; 331(7522):932–8.

[44] Feringa HH, Bax JJ, Boersma E, et al. High-dose beta-blockers and tight heart rate control reduce myocardial ischemia and troponin T release in vascular surgery patients. Circulation 2006;114(Suppl 1): I344–9.

[45] Poldermans D, Bax JJ, Schouten O, et al. Should major vascular surgery be delayed because of preoperative cardiac testing in intermediate-risk patients receiving beta-blocker therapy with tight heart rate control? J Am Coll Cardiol 2006;48(5):964–9.

[46] Devereaux PJ, Yang H, Guyatt GH, et al. Rationale, design, and organization of the PeriOperative ISchemic Evaluation (POISE) trial: a randomized controlled trial of metoprolol versus placebo in patients undergoing noncardiac surgery. Am Heart J 2006;152(2):223–30.

[47] Wijeysundera DN, Naik JS, Beattie WS. Alpha-2 adrenergic agonists to prevent perioperative cardiovascular complications: a meta-analysis. Am J Med 2003;114(9):742–52.

[48] Wallace AW, Galindez D, Salahieh A, et al. Effect of clonidine on cardiovascular morbidity and mortality after noncardiac surgery. Anesthesiology 2004; 101(2):284–93.

[49] Kapoor AS, Kanji H, Buckingham J, et al. Strength of evidence for perioperative use of statins to reduce cardiovascular risk: systematic review of controlled studies. BMJ 2006;333(7579):1149–55.

[50] Durazzo AE, Machado FS, Ikeoka DT, et al. Reduction in cardiovascular events after vascular surgery with atorvastatin: a randomized trial. J Vasc Surg 2004;39(5):967–75 [discussion: 975–6].

[51] Feringa HH, Schouten O, Karagiannis SE, et al. Intensity of statin therapy in relation to myocardial ischemia, troponin T release, and clinical cardiac outcome in patients undergoing major vascular surgery. J Am Coll Cardiol 2007;50(17):1649–56.

[52] Schouten O, Hoeks SE, Welten GM, et al. Effect of statin withdrawal on frequency of cardiac events after vascular surgery. Am J Cardiol 2007;100(2):316–20.

[53] Schouten O, Kertai MD, Bax JJ, et al. Safety of perioperative statin use in high-risk patients undergoing major vascular surgery. Am J Cardiol 2005;95(5): 658–60.

[54] Schouten O, Poldermans D, Visser L, et al. Fluvastatin and bisoprolol for the reduction of perioperative cardiac mortality and morbidity in high-risk patients undergoing non-cardiac surgery: rationale and design of the DECREASE-IV study. Am Heart J 2004;148(6):1047–52.

[55] De Decker K, Jorens PG, Van Schil P. Cardiac complications after noncardiac thoracic surgery: an evidence-based current review. Ann Thorac Surg 2003;75(4):1340–8.

[56] Shrivastava V, Nyawo B, Dunning J, et al. Is there a role for prophylaxis against atrial fibrillation for patients undergoing lung surgery? Interact Cardiovasc Thorac Surg 2004;3(4):656–62.

[57] Ulicny KS Jr, Schmelzer V, Flege JB Jr, et al. Concomitant cardiac and pulmonary operation: the role of cardiopulmonary bypass. Ann Thorac Surg 1992;54(2):289–95.

[58] Rosalion A, Woodford NW, Clarke CP, et al. Concomitant coronary revascularization and resection of lung cancer. Aust N Z J Surg 1993;63(5):336–40.

[59] Yokoyama T, Derrick MJ, Lee AW. Cardiac operation with associated pulmonary resection. J Thorac Cardiovasc Surg 1993;105(5):912–6 [discussion: 916–7].

[60] Terzi A, Furlan G, Magnanelli G, et al. Lung resections concomitant to coronary artery bypass grafting. Eur J Cardiothorac Surg 1994;8(11):580–4.

[61] Thomas P, Giudicelli R, Guillen JC, et al. Is lung cancer surgery justified in patients with coronary artery disease? Eur J Cardiothorac Surg 1994;8(6): 287–91 [discussion: 292].

[62] Miller DL, Orszulak TA, Pairolero PC, et al. Combined operation for lung cancer and cardiac disease. Ann Thorac Surg 1994;58(4):989–93 [discussion: 993–4].

[63] Johnson JA, Landreneau RJ, Boley TM, et al. Should pulmonary lesions be resected at the time of open heart surgery? Am Surg 1996;62(4):300–3.

[64] Rao V, Todd TR, Weisel RD, et al. Results of combined pulmonary resection and cardiac operation. Ann Thorac Surg 1996;62(2):342–6 [discussion: 346–7].

[65] Voets AJ, Joesoef KS, van Teeffelen ME. Synchronously occurring lung cancer (stages I-II) and coronary artery disease: concomitant versus staged surgical approach. Eur J Cardiothorac Surg 1997; 12(5):713–7.

[66] Danton MH, Anikin VA, McManus KG, et al. Simultaneous cardiac surgery with pulmonary resection: presentation of series and review of literature. Eur J Cardiothorac Surg 1998;13(6): 667–72.

[67] Mariani MA, van Boven WJ, Duurkens VA, et al. Combined off-pump coronary surgery and right lung resections through midline sternotomy. Ann Thorac Surg 2001;71(4):1343–4.

[68] Ambrogi V, Pompeo E, Elia S, et al. The impact of cardiovascular comorbidity on the outcome of surgery for stage I and II non-small-cell lung cancer. Eur J Cardiothorac Surg 2003;23(5): 811–7.

[69] Dyszkiewicz W, Jemielity MM, Piwkowski CT, et al. Simultaneous lung resection for cancer and myocardial revascularization without cardiopulmonary bypass (off-pump coronary artery bypass grafting). Ann Thorac Surg 2004;77(3): 1023–7.

[70] Schoenmakers MC, van Boven WJ, van den Bosch J, et al. Comparison of on-pump or off-pump coronary artery revascularization with lung resection. Ann Thorac Surg 2007;84(2):504–9.

ELSEVIER
SAUNDERS

Thorac Surg Clin 18 (2008) 61–69

THORACIC
SURGERY
CLINICS

Predicting the Need for Intensive Care Following Lung Resection

Simon Jordan, MD, FRCS[a,b], Timothy W. Evans, MD, PhD[a,b,*]

[a]*Department of Thoracic Surgery, Royal Brompton Hospital, Sydney Street, London SW3 6NP, UK*
[b]*Department of Intensive Care Medicine, Imperial College School of Medicine, Royal Brompton Hospital, Sydney Street, London SW3 6NP, UK*

The nature and frequency of lung resection procedures

The use of screening techniques, such as computed and positron emission tomography, in patients thought to be at high risk of developing primary lung tumors is increasing. These can be successful in identifying early stage lesions, resulting in potential resection rates in the order of 95% [1]. Consequently, the number of patients presenting for such surgery is likely to increase. Presently, national and international registries suggest that considerable international and intranational variation exists in clinical practice. This can be illustrated by the institutional pneumonectomy rate in Norway, which varies from 45% to 9.5% of lung resections [2]. The overall resection rate of 16.4% reported is much higher than that reported in the United Kingdom [3], but may be lower than rates in the United States. Variations in Europe are considerable, reported as ranging from 7% in Teesside, UK to 24% in Varese, Italy.

Despite overall improvements in outcome [4], pulmonary resection for malignancy is still associated with significant morbidity [5] likely to necessitate protracted periods of postoperative intensive care. As populations age and comorbidities in those presenting for surgery increase in number and complexity, this requirement is likely to rise, influenced in part by changes in clinical decision making. Both anatomic and nonanatomic sub lobar resections have been performed in selected patients to preserve lung parenchyma. However, randomized trial data show that this is associated with a greater incidence of local recurrence and reduced survival. Anticipating, and preferably predicting, which patients undergoing thoracic surgery will require intensive care postoperatively therefore assumes considerable clinical significance, and has implications for resource provision and utilization.

Mortality following lung resection

Major advances in thoracic surgery and anesthesia, and in the delivery of postoperative care, have led to reductions in postoperative mortality following lung resection. Estimates of death associated with such surgery, published in the early 1990s, vary from 2% to 12% [6,7]. More recent reviews still indicate 30-day mortality of up to 5% to 10%, with higher rates expected for complex procedures and in the setting of pneumonectomy performed for benign disease [5]. Single center series have revealed lower (in the order of 4.8%, [8]) or comparable (7.5%, [9]) mortality rates. Furthermore, recent attempts to identify more precisely in-hospital mortality following lung resection have emerged from national and international sources. Examination of a nationally representative thoracic surgical database receiving entries from June 2002 to July 2005 demonstrates that of 15,183 original patients, 338 (2.2%) died during the same hospital admission [10]. Similarly, the European Thoracic Surgery system receiving data

Work is supported in part by the John Moulton Trust.

* Corresponding author. Department of Thoracic Surgery, Royal Brompton Hospital, Sydney Street, London SW3 6NP, UK.

E-mail address: t.evans@rbht.nhs.uk (T.W. Evans).

1547-4127/08/$ - see front matter
doi:10.1016/j.thorsurg.2007.11.003

from 27 units in 14 countries indicates that of 3,426 adult patients undergoing a first lung resection for whom mortality data were available, 66 (1.9%) died within the same hospital admission [11].

Morbidity following lung resection

Interpretation of published data

Data concerning morbidity after thoracic surgery are relatively plentiful, but difficult to interpret, especially in the context of the requirement for intensive care unit (ICU) admission in the postoperative period. Thus, international variation in patient selection may be relevant in leading to exclusion or inclusion of those with pre-existing comorbidities. The availability of resources may result in only those with early disease coming to surgical resection. The frequent observation that outcome is poorer after pneumonectomy may be because such patients have more extensive cancers, additional morbidity associated with the complications of the pneumonectomy space, or worse survival because of inadequate postoperative lung capacity and function. By contrast, inadequate screening facilities could lead paradoxically to patients presenting for operative resection with advanced disease states, thereby influencing both mortality and morbidity. A lack of postoperative or critical care resources could similarly influence outcomes adversely.

Conditions associated with adverse outcome

Conditions associated with adverse outcome can be divided broadly into conditions afflicting the lung directly and extra pulmonary pathologies (Box 1). Complications may occur as a result of technical complications of surgery itself (eg, bronchopleural fistula or BPF), those which may be related to the underlying condition or primary pathology (eg, pulmonary thrombo embolism, the incidence of which is increased in patients with malignancy), and conditions which may or may not be related to either (eg, postoperative pneumonia).

Box 1. Conditions associated with adverse outcome following lung resection

Pulmonary
- Pulmonary fibrosis
- Poor lung function
- Recent smoking

Nonpulmonary
- Age (greater than 70 years old)
- Preoperative chemotherapy
- Obesity
- Cardiac disease
- Hepatorenal dysfunction

Postoperative pulmonary complications

Acute lung injury (ALI), acute respiratory distress syndrome (ARDS), and postpenumonectomy pulmonary edema (PPE) are all postoperative pulmonary complications (Box 2). In terms of adverse effects on mortality, PPE is the most significant complication of pneumonectomy or lobectomy, developing in between 1% (wedge resection), 2% to 3% (lobectomy, bilobectomy), and 5% to 7% (pneumonectomy) of patients, and with an associated mortality in the order of 40% to 60% [8,9,12,13]. In its extreme form, PPE follows a clinical and histopathologic course indistinguishable from ALI and its extreme manifestation ARDS, and is said to be the biggest single cause of postoperative mortality [13]. ICU admission is mandatory for the care of such patients, but predicting the onset of ALI and ARDS is difficult.

Pre- and perioperative factors associated with lung injury, aside from the extent of resection, are said to include perioperative fluid overload [14,15], although the high protein content of the alveolar edema fluid in patients with PPE, and the frequent delay in presentation to the third

Box 2. Complications of pulmonary resection

Pulmonary
- ARDS, ALI, PPE
- Bronchopleural fistula
- Empyema
- Postoperative pneumonia

Nonpulmonary
- Thromboembolism
- Arryhthmia
- Acute myocardial infarction
- Cerebro-vascular accident
- Hemorrhage
- Renal failure
- Sepsis or multiorgan failure

postoperative day or beyond, both mitigate against this theory. Impaired lymphatic drainage through disruption of ipsilateral lymphatic drainage channels incurred during lobectomy and pneumonectomy may be relevant, especially as it is now standard practice in many units to perform systematic nodal dissection during surgery for pulmonary malignancy. However, studies involving lymphatic injection of dye, and those attempting to associate the extent of PPE with the side of surgery and relationship to the lymphatic duct, have provided conflicting results [16,17]. It is probably reasonable to assume that lymphatic disruption may play some role in the clinical severity of PPE, although it is unlikely to be responsible for its onset alone. The duration of surgery seems to be unimportant [18], but the influence of one lung ventilation may be more relevant. Studies suggesting that conventional tidal volumes delivered to patients with pre-existing lung injury may propagate inflammation and disseminate it into the systemic circulation [19] have led to questions regarding the optimum means of delivering one lung ventilation. High tidal volumes or peak inspiratory pressures administered to a lung with preoperative, possibly smoking-related, impairments in compliance, airways resistance, and the like, may lead to baro- or volotrauma. An associated requirement for increased inspired oxygen concentrations may lead to cytotoxicity. In a single center retrospective study of 170 patients undergoing pneumonectomy, postoperative respiratory complications of all kinds (PPE, BPF, pulmonary thromboembolism) leading to respiratory failure (defined as the requirement for mechanical ventilation of more than 48 hours) was associated with the application of larger intraoperative tidal volumes (8.7 mL/kg median), compared with patients who did not (6.7 mL/kg) [20].

In summary, the type and intensity of mechanical ventilation applied during one lung anesthesia may contribute to the development of PPE, but a causal link has not been established. Further exploration of the mechanisms underlying PPE may be possible using noninvasive systems. Thus, after lobectomy, the concentration in exhaled breath condensate of proinflammatory moieties including leukotriene B4, hydrogen peroxide, and hydrogen ions have been shown to rise significantly [21].

Bronchopleural fistula

The incidence of BPF seems to occur in between 4% (all cases) and 8% (after pneumonectomy) of patients [9,22,23]. Its development is significantly associated with resection for benign disease, lower preoperative forced expiratory volume in the first second of expiration (FEV_1) and diffusing capacity of the lung for carbon monoxide (DLCO), right sided pneumonectomy, bronchial stump reinforcement, completion pneumonectomy, timing of chest tube removal, increased intravenous fluid administration in the first 12 hours, and the need for blood transfusion or mechanical ventilation.

Empyema

In a single center series [22], empyema complicated some 5.7% of cases and was also predicted by univariate analysis in association with surgery for benign disease, low preoperative hemoglobin, FEV_1 and DLCO, right sided pneumonectomy, bronchial stump reinforcement, completion pneumonectomy, timing of chest tube removal, and the need for blood transfusion or mechanical ventilation.

Pneumonia

Postoperative pneumonia (POP) is a life threatening complication of lung resection. In a single center study of over 150 subjects recruited over 6 months [24], bronchial colonization was identified in samples obtained perioperatively in a surprisingly large proportion of cases (22%). The incidence of POP was 25%, the majority of cases being microbiologically identified. Species most commonly isolated were *Haemophilus influenzae*, Streptococci, and more rarely *Pseudomonas* and *Serratia*. POP was more common in the colonized population. Patients with POP needed support with noninvasive or invasive mechanical ventilation more frequently than those with no infection. POP was also associated with longer ICU and hospital lengths of stay. Factors associated with the incidence of POP were pre-existing chronic obstructive pulmonary disease, the extent of resection, male sex, and the presence of intraoperative colonization. Others have found the incidence of pneumonia to be lower (eg, 6.4%) and to be more commonly the consequence of Gram-negative infection (94% of cases) [9].

Acute interstitial pneumonia (AIP) has been described in 2% of more than 800 patients undergoing resection of primary lung cancer. In all cases, radiologic changes appeared within 1 week of surgery, with most patients requiring mechanical ventilatory support. Right sided tumors, pneumonectomy, preoperative radiation or chemotherapy, blood transfusion, and intraoperative complications were identified as independent risk factors and the associated mortality was over 50% [25]. Differentiating AIP from ALI or ARDS may prove to be difficult in practice.

Postoperative nonpulmonary complications

Pulmonary thromboembolism

The literature dealing with the incidence and management of acute pulmonary thromboembolism (PTE) after resection of lung cancer is limited, although patients are at increased risk by virtue of underlying malignancy and immobility in the postoperative period, in addition to the influence of active respiratory or cardiac pathologies, obesity or age (older than 60 years) [26]. The incidence of PTE has been calculated to be around 1%, and ranked eighth in frequency of pulmonary complications [9]. General preventative measures should include the use of mechanical devices (eg, graduated compression or antiembolus stockings), low molecular weight heparin, avoidance of dehydration, and early postoperative mobility. Small series suggest that patients with pulmonary embolism after surgery for lung cancer can be treated aggressively with anticoagulants with or without fibrinolytics, or can even undergo pulmonary embolectomy on cardiopulmonary bypass, without excessive risk of bleeding complications [27].

Cardiovascular complications of lung resection

Cardiovascular complications include symptomatic arrhythmias requiring treatment, acute myocardial infarction, and stroke. The presence of coronary artery disease increases the risk of nonfatal myocardial infarction or death within 30 days of noncardiac surgery, although data relating specifically to patients undergoing thoracic surgery are sparse. However, in an investigation of nearly 400 patients undergoing lung resection, nearly 13% (n = 24) died of cardiovascular and respiratory causes (acute respiratory failure, pneumonia, pulmonary embolism, acute pulmonary edema, acute myocardial ischemia, or stroke). These 24 patients had a higher frequency of pre-existing coronary artery disease or heart failure, predicted postoperative FEV_1 less than 1,000 mL, exertional dyspnea, and 30-day operative cardiopulmonary complications [28].

Influence of preoperative conditions on the incidence of perioperative complications

Pulmonary fibrosis

Pulmonary fibrosis is associated with an increased risk of lung malignancy [29]. Relatively few studies, however, have investigated the risks associated with pre-existing lung fibrosis in patients undergoing lung resection. In a single center Japanese study, 7.5% of those operated upon had idiopathic pulmonary fibrosis (IPF), but suffered pulmonary morbidity and mortality rates in excess of those without (26% versus 9.1%). The 5-year survival was 43% among patients with IPF (versus 64.2%), although disease-free survival was similar [30]. In a second, smaller study of patients with stage 1 cancer, no early postoperative deaths occurred, but a second malignancy developed in 36% of those who ultimately died. A significant number of patients succumbed eventually to exacerbations of IPF, although whether these were triggered by surgery is unclear [31]. Finally, in a study comparing outcome in 22 patients with pulmonary fibrosis with over 900 patients without undergoing lung resection, operative mortality was higher in the IPF group (17% versus 3.1%), as were the incidences of PPE (21% versus 3.7%) and hospital length of stay [32].

These data suggest that pre-existing pulmonary fibrosis is associated with poorer outcome after lung resection. Whether this is because of the associated impairment in lung function or is specific to IPF is unclear. Moreover, the increased incidence of malignancy in such patients, and the poor prognosis of patients undergoing ICU admission with lung fibrosis per se, suggest that careful preoperative evaluation and perioperative management are required to optimize surgical outcome.

Smoking and the influence of smoking cessation

The benefits of smoking cessation in preventing postoperative pulmonary complications remain controversial, in that some studies have demonstrated benefit, but others have revealed a paradoxical increase in complications in those quitting smoking only a few weeks or days before surgery. In part, this may reflect difficulties in categorizing patients accurately into nonsmokers, past quitters of varying month's duration, recent quitters, and ongoing smokers. Nevertheless, in comparing recent (defined as less than 2 months) quitters with ongoing smokers in a relatively large scale study of over 300 patients undergoing resection for primary or metastatic cancer, no difference in pulmonary complications emerged postoperatively (23% for both groups), although this incidence was considerably higher than that for nonsmokers (8%) and past quitters (19%)

[33]. Others have confirmed that postoperative pulmonary complications gradually decrease in frequency over time after quitting; providing the period was 5 to 8 weeks or longer [34]. The crucial period seems to be around 1 month; in performing multivariate analysis on relevant variables in over 250 patients undergoing pneumonectomy, only the timing of smoking cessation (1 month or sooner before operation) was a significant predictor of a major pulmonary event.

Therefore, there seems to be no evidence of a paradoxical increase in pulmonary complications among those who quit smoking within 2 months of undergoing surgery. Moreover, those who continue to smoke up to 1 month before their operation are at significant risk of pulmonary complications.

Preoperative chemotherapy

The administration of neoadjuvant chemotherapy before resection of nonsmall cell lung cancer has been suggested to increase survival, mainly in the early stage. In some cases neoadjuvant chemotherapy may downstage a patient's disease and render them potentially operable. Risks of postoperative complications after chemotherapy and surgery remain controversial, however. In an early publication, an increased risk was perceived, of 11% for all pneumonectomies and lobectomies, and 23% for right pneumonectomy, with complications occurring in 38% of cases [35]. In a more recent series of over 100 patients treated with varying induction chemotherapies (mainly cisplatin with vinorelbine or gemicitabine), postoperative mortality was low (two patients), with no deaths after lobectomy. However, complications occurred in 29% of patients (33 of 114), usually infectious pneumonia and anemia requiring transfusion. In univariate and multivariate analyses, preoperative FEV_1, hemoglobin, and partial pressure of oxygen in the alveoli (PaO_2) were not associated with morbidity [36]. In many series, chemotherapeutic regimens have not been standardized, but the European Organization for Research and Treatment of Cancer (EORTC) 08941 phase-III trial of surgical resection versus radiotherapy in proven stage IIIA-N2 nonsmall cell lung cancer employed a platinum-based induction chemotherapy. Subjects proceeded to surgery after an objective response. Operative 30-day mortality in the 167 subjects randomized to the surgical arm was 4.0% [37]. Postoperative complications included pneumonia, respiratory insufficiency, arrhythmias, air leak, cardiac decompensation, empyema and broncho-pleural fistula.

Thus, while early concerns were raised about the possible adverse effects of adjuvant therapy upon outcome after subsequent surgical resection, the EORTC trial at least yielded acceptable rates of morbidity and mortality.

Preoperative prediction of the need for postoperative intensive care

Routine admission to intensive care after lung resection

The influence of the elective ICU admission on outcome after major lung resection has been investigated only rarely. In a single study [38], early outcome was compared in a center managing all patients in a dedicated ward—resorting to ICU only for the management of complications requiring invasive assisted ventilation—to that in a second center that electively transferred high risk cases to ICU immediately after operation. Nearly 100 pairs of patients matched for severity were compared. Trends toward reduced total morbidity (23% versus 35%), cardiovascular (13.5% versus 23%), and pulmonary complication rates (9.3% versus 18%) were observed, but at the cost of longer postoperative hospital stay (11.5 versus 9.7 days) in patients admitted electively to the ICU. Mortality did not differ (7.3% versus 7.3%). While elective postoperative ICU admission did not show a clear-cut outcome benefit over management in a dedicated ward, these data again indicate a relatively high incidence of postoperative complications in this population and re-emphasizes the need for careful preoperative selection. This may be based upon general and pulmonary considerations.

Nonpulmonary predictive factors for poor outcome (and therefore potential intensive care unit admission); large scale studies

Two large studies have attempted to model predictive factors for poor outcome. The European Thoracic Surgery Database project [11] applied logistic regression to a random sample of 60% of cases to identify preoperative factors associated with in-hospital mortality and to build a model of risk. The resulting model was tested on the remaining 40% of a total of almost 3,500 patients. Within the data used for model development, dyspnoea (according to the Medical Research Council classification), American Society of Anaesthesiologists (ASA) score, class of procedure, and age were found to be significantly associated with in-hospital death in multivariate analysis. The logistic model developed for all diagnoses performed well at low risk, underestimated mortality at medium risk, and overestimated mortality at high risk.

A second large-scale study [10] in over 15,000 patients developed a risk model for in-hospital death, again employing a sub set of data (two thirds of patients) subsequently validated on the remainder. Factors significantly associated with the occurrence of in-hospital death in multivariate analysis were again age, sex, dyspnea score, ASA score, performance status classification, priority of surgery, diagnosis group, procedure class, and comorbid disease. The model was reliable for both the training and test sets of data.

In establishing the need for ICU admission in the postoperative period, age is therefore relevant. For those older than 70 years, the mortality from reported series for lobectomy is between 4% and 7%, and for pneumonectomy averages 14% [4]. These rates are higher than for patients under 70 years old and the differential between the mortality of pneumonectomy and lobectomy is larger in elderly patients when compared with younger patients, but these differences may be more a function of comorbidity than age alone [39]. Information is limited on the mortality rates for lung cancer resection in the very elderly (older than 80 years) but suggest that the very elderly can tolerate lobectomy. As with any planned major operation, especially in a population predisposed to atherosclerotic cardiovascular disease by cigarette smoking, a preoperative cardiovascular risk assessment should be performed [40].

Pulmonary predictive factors for poor outcome (and therefore potential intensive care unit admission)

While lung function and exercise capacity decrease within the first few months following lung cancer resection, they may recover to some extent thereafter [41]. There are few data concerning the immediate postoperative period. Thus, ideally, preoperative assessment would permit the identification of those at high risk for perioperative (pulmonary) complications and therefore the need for ICU admission. Moreover, this would permit more effective counseling of patients concerning treatment options and associated risks to inform decision-making. Both the British Thoracic Society [42] and American College of Chest Physicians have produced guidelines for investigating patients for lung cancer surgery, but these were based on relatively old studies.

Estimations of predicted postoperative (ppo) lung function have been made using different methods. Each is designed to quantify the functioning lung that would be lost because of surgical resection of tumor. Ventilation and perfusion scans, quantitative computed tomography, and merely counting the number of segments to be resected seem to provide similar estimates of ppo lung function. Recommended approaches use a radionuclide perfusion scan with Tc-labeled macroaggregates of albumin to estimate the ppo FEV_1 and DLCO after pneumonectomy, and the number of segments remaining for postlobectomy values [42]. The percentage of ppo values for FEV_1 and DLCO are routinely used instead of absolute values.

How useful are such investigations in determining the need for intensive care admission? A recently published study [43] of over 100 patients (hospital mortality rate 3%, major complication rate 22%) found that all lung function values were better predictors of poor surgical outcome when expressed as a percentage of the predicted value, and that a preoperative FEV_1 of 47% predicted resulted in the most useful positive and negative predictive probabilities (0.90 and 0.67, respectively). Such thresholds have been investigated with specific reference to ICU admission in only one published study [44]. Of 170 patients undergoing lung resection, 52 (30%) needed intensive care postoperatively: 21 (12%) for less than 24 hours and 31 (18%) for more, for which group the average length of stay was 11.3 days. There was no significant difference between the patient groups at ICU admission in terms of median severity of illness (acute physiology and chronic health evaluation or APACHE II) scores, gas exchange (PaO_2, or fraction inspired oxygen [FiO_2], 441 versus 364 mm Hg), nor in estimated postoperative absolute (1.62 versus 1.31 l) or predicted percentage (61.8% versus 44.3%) FEV_1.

These data illustrate three points. First, in this study as in others a major clinical problem encountered postoperatively in those needing a protracted stay (ie, longer than 24 hours) is impaired gas exchange. Thus, mean PaO_2 to FiO_2 ratio at admission for those requiring an extended ICU stay was 290 mm Hg, fulfilling the American-European Consensus Conference defining criteria for acute lung injury, and 4% of patients undergoing surgery fulfilled the defining gas exchange criteria for ARDS [45]. Of the variables cited as relevant to the development of PPE, in this study no relationship emerged between operative time, the presence of preoperative respiratory impairment (evidenced by spirometry), and the extent of resection, predicted postoperative FEV_1 and the requirement for protracted ICU admission. In reality, the pathophysiology of lung injury after pulmonary resection is likely to be multifactorial in etiology and a composite measure of pulmonary dysfunction might provide a more robust method of predicting the need for protracted ventilation and ICU care.

Second, the data do indicate that patients requiring a prolonged ICU stay have significantly higher APACHE II scores at admission than those who do not. Although the score comprises many different components, the increased requirement for renal support, nitrous oxide therapy, and tracheostomy in the extended stay group reinforces the impression that patients are generally less well, and not merely from the respiratory viewpoint.

Finally, patients undergoing pulmonary resection for suspected malignancy clearly consume considerable ICU resources. In 12% of cases in this study the requirement was relatively modest, amounting to little more than an extended period of after surgical recovery. By contrast, in 17% of cases a prolonged stay was needed (mean 11 days) in whom the average cost was nearly £24,000 (approximately $48,000 USD). It is important to note that the cohort of patients studied seemed to compare favorably with previously reported series. Indeed, the mortality rate of 2.3% betters many previously reported [4,10,11], and the incidence of ARDS (2%) was lower than others previously published [45].

Summary

On the basis of the evidence available, the authors would suggest a decision making algorithm to determine the need for ICU admission postoperatively similar to that shown in Fig. 1. First, patients should quit smoking at least 1 month and preferably 2 months before surgery. Those over the age of 70 years should receive elective ICU admission. Second, those at increased risk of general anesthesia, as judged by ASA and performance status scores and cardiovascular risk assessment, should be prebooked into the ICU in the postoperative period. A ppo FEV_1 of less than 44% should warrant additional monitoring rather than mandate ICU admission. Pre-existing fibrotic lung disease mandates ICU admission. Third, perioperatively, protective (low tidal volume) ventilatory strategies should be applied during one lung ventilation. Patients undergoing one lung ventilation, and especially those undergoing extensive lymphatic dissection, should be monitored closely for signs of ALI in the first 5 days postoperatively. This, together with any indication of postoperative complications such as POP, BPF or empyema, should mandate immediate transfer to the ICU.

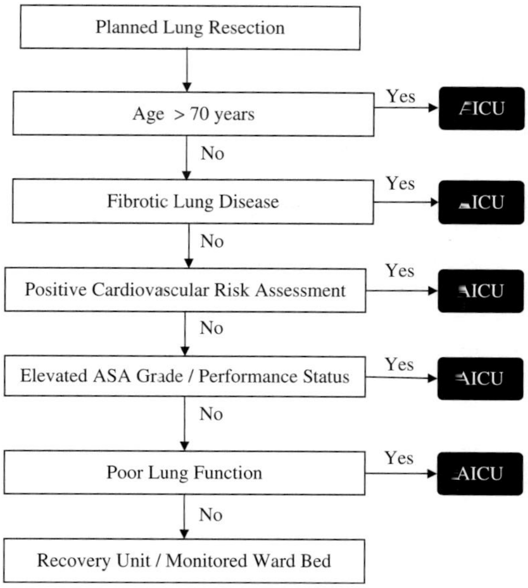

Fig. 1. Selection criteria for elective admission to intensive care following lung resection.

References

[1] Pastorino U, Bellomi M, Landoni C, et al. Early lung-cancer detection with spiral CT and positron emission tomography in heavy smokers: 2-year results. Lancet 2003;362:593–7.

[2] Strand TE, Rostad H, Moller B, et al. Survival after resection for primary lung cancer: a population-based study of 3211 resected patients. Thorax 2006;61:710–5.

[3] Laroche C, Wells F, Coulden R, et al. Improving surgical resection rate in lung cancer. Thorax 1998; 53(6):445–9.

[4] Damhuis RA, Schutte PR. Resection rate and postoperative mortality in 7,899 patients with lung cancer. Eur Respir J 1996;9(1):7–10.

[5] Klemperer J, Ginsberg RJ. Morbidity and mortality after pneumonectomy. Chest Surg Clin N Am 1999; 9(3):515–25.

[6] Wada H, Nakamura T, Nakamoto K, et al. Thirty day operative mortality for thoracotomy in lung cancer. J Thorac Cardiovasc Surg 1998;115:70–3.
[7] Romano PS, Mark DH. Patient and hospital characteristics related to in hospital mortality after lung cancer resection. Chest 1992;101:1332–7.
[8] Kutlu CA, Williams EA, Evans TW, et al. Acute lung injury and acute respiratory distress syndrome after pulmonary resection. Ann Thorac Surg 2000; 69:376–80.
[9] Stephan F, Boucheseiche S, Hollande J, et al. Pulmonary complications following lung resection. Chest 2000;118(5):1263–70.
[10] Falcoz PE, Conti M, Brouchet L, et al. The thoracic surgery scoring system (Thoracoscore): risk model for in-hospital death in 15,183 patients requiring thoracic surgery. J Thorac Cardiovasc Surg 2007; 133(2):325–32.
[11] Berrisford R, Brunelli A, Rocco G, et al. European thoracic surgery database project: modeling the risk of in hospital death following lung resection. Eur J Cardiothorac Surg 2005;28:306–11.
[12] Ruffini E, Parola A, Papalia E, et al. Frequency and mortality of acute lung injury and acute respiratory distress syndrome after pulmonary resection for bronchogenic carcinoma. Eur J Cardiothorac Surg 2001;20(1):30–6.
[13] Dulu A, Pastores S, Park B, et al. Prevelence and mortality of acute lung injury and ARDS after lung resection. Chest 2006;130(1):73–8.
[14] Patel RL, Townsend ER, Fountain SW. Elective pneumonectomy: factors associated with morbidity and operative mortality. Ann Thorac Surg 1992;54: 84–8.
[15] Lee E, Little AG, Hsu WH, et al. Effect of pneumonectomy on extravascular lung water in dogs. J Surg Res 1985;38:568–73.
[16] Turnage WS, Lunn JJ. Post pneumonectomy pulmonary edema: a restrospective analysis of associated variables. Chest 1993;103:1646–50.
[17] Waller DA, Gebitekin C, Saunders NR, et al. Non cardiogenic pulmonary oedema complicating lung resection. Ann Thorac Surg 1993;55:140–3.
[18] Zeldin RA, Normandin D, Landtwing D, et al. Post pneumonectomy pulmonary edema. J Thorac Cardiovasc Surg 1984;87:359–65.
[19] Ranieri VM, Suter PM, Tortorella C, et al. Effect of mechanical ventilation on inflammatory mediators in patients with acute respiratory distress syndrome: a randomized controlled trial. JAMA 1999;282(1): 54–61.
[20] Frenadez Perez ER, Keegan MT, Brown DR, et al. Intraoperative tidal volume as a risk factor for respiratory failure after pneumonectomy. Anesthesiology 2006;105:14–8.
[21] Moloney ED, Mumby SE, Gojdocsi K, et al. Exhaled breath condensate detects markers of pulmonary inflammation after cardiothoracic surgery. Am J Respir Crit Care Med 2004;169(1):64–9.
[22] Deschamps C, Bernard A, Nichols FC, et al. Empyema and bronchopleural fistula after pneumonectomy; factors affecting incidence. Ann Thorac Surg 2001;72(1):243–7.
[23] Sirbu H, Busch T, Alecksic I, et al. Bronchopleural fistula in the surgery of non small cell lung cancer: incidence, risk factors and management. Ann Thorac Cardiovasc Surg 2001;7(6):330–6.
[24] Schussler O, Alifano M, Dermine H, et al. Post operative pneumonia after lung resection. Am J Respir Crit Care Med 2006;173(10):1161–9.
[25] Muraoka M, Tagawa T, Akamine S, et al. Acute interstitial pneumonia following surgery for primary lung cancer. Eur J Cardiothorac Surg 2006;30(4): 657–62.
[26] Hill J, Treasure T. Reducing the risk of venous thromboembolism (deep vein thrombosis and pulmonary embolism) in inpatients having surgery; summary of NICE guidance. BMJ 2007;334:1053–4.
[27] Sakuragi T, Sakao Y, Furukawa K, et al. Successful management of acute pulmonary embolism after surgery for lung cancer. Eur J Cardiothorac Surg 2003;24(4):580–7.
[28] Volpino P, Cangemi R, Fiori E, et al. Risk of mortality from cardiovascular and respiratory causes in patients with chronic obstructive pulmonary disease submitted to follow-up after lung resection for non-small cell lung cancer. J Cardiovasc Surg (Torino) 2007;48(3):375–83.
[29] Hubbard R, Venn A, Lewis S. Lung cancer and cryptogenic fibrosing alveolitis. A population-based cohort study. Am J Respir Crit Care Med 2000; 161(1):5–8.
[30] Kawasaki H, Nagai K, Yoshida J, et al. Postoperative morbidity, mortality and survival in lung cancer associated with idiopathic pulmonary fibrosis. J Surg Oncol 2002;81:33–7.
[31] Fujimoto T, Okazaki T, Matsukura T, et al. Operation for lung cancer in patients with idiopathic pulmonary fibrosis: surgical contra indication? Ann Thorac Surg 2003;76:1674–8.
[32] Kumar P, Goldstraw P, Yamada K, et al. Pulmonary fibrosis and lung cancer: risk and benefit analysis of pulmonary resection. J Thorac Cardiovasc Surg 2003;125(6):1321–7.
[33] Barrera R, Shi W, Amar D, et al. Smoking and timing of cessation: impact on pulmonary complications after thoracotomy. Chest 2005;127:1873–83.
[34] Nakagawa M, Tanaka H, Tsukuma H, et al. Relationship between the duration of postoperative smoke free period and the incidence of post operative pulmonary complications after pulmonary surgery. Chest 2001;120:705–10.
[35] Martin J, Ginsberg RJ, Abolhoda A, et al. A Morbidity and mortality after neoadjuvant therapy for lung cancer: the risks of right pneumonectomy. Ann Thorac Surg 2001;72(4):1149–54.
[36] Perrot E, Guibert B, Mulsant P, et al. Preoperative chemotherapy does not increase complications after

nonsmall cell lung cancer resection. Ann Thorac Surg 2005;80(6):423–7.

[37] Van Schil P, Van Meerbeeck J, Kramer G, et al. Morbidity and mortality in the surgery arm of EORTC 08941 trial. Eur Respir J 2005;26(2): 192–7.

[38] Brunelli A, Pieretti P, Al Refai M, et al. Elective intensive care alter luna resection: a multicentric propensity-matched comparison of outcome. Interact Cardiovasc Thorac Surg 2005;4(6): 609–13.

[39] Yellin A, Hill LR, Lieberman Y. Pulmonary resections in patients over 70 years of age. Isr J Med Sci 1985;21:833–40.

[40] Eagle KA, Brundage BH, Chaitman BR, et al. Guidelines for perioperative cardiovascular evaluation for noncardiac surgery: report of the American College of Cardiology/American Heart Association Task Force on Practice Guidelines. J Am Coll Cardiol 1996;27:910–48.

[41] Nezu K, Kushibe K, Tojo T, et al. Recovery and limitation of exercise capacity after lung resection for lung cancer. Chest 1998;113:1511–6.

[42] British Thoracic Society. BTS guidelines: guidelines on the selection of patients with lung cancer for surgery. Thorax 2001;56:89–108.

[43] Win T, Jackson A, Sharples L. Relationship between pulmonary function and lung cancer surgical outcome. Eur Respir J 2005;25(4):594–9.

[44] Melley DD, Thomson EM, Page SP, et al. Incidence, duration and causes of intensive care unit admission following pulmonary resection for malignancy. Intensive Care Med 2006;32:1419–22.

[45] Jordan S, Mitchell JA, Quinlan GJ, et al. The pathogenesis of lung injury following pulmonary resection. Eur Respir J 2000;15:790–9.

ELSEVIER
SAUNDERS

Thorac Surg Clin 18 (2008) 71–80

THORACIC
SURGERY
CLINICS

Risks of Neoadjuvant Chemotherapy and Radiation Therapy

Georgios Stamatis, FETCS

Department of Thoracic Surgery and Endoscopy, Ruhrlandklinik Essen-Heidhausen, Tüschenerweg 40, 45239 Essen, Germany

Lung cancer remains one of the most common malignancies and is the leading cause of cancer-related deaths in Europe and North America [1,2]. Because of the poor long-term prognosis and the overall 5-year survival rate of less than 15%, the development of optimized treatment approaches remains a continuing challenge [3]. In non–small-cell lung cancer (NSCLC), the main curative therapeutic approach is surgery for early stages IA to IIB. However, early stages constitute only 20% to 25% of all NSCLC patients, whereas the majority of patients initially present with locally advanced stages IIIA/IIIB or even with metastasized disease. Only small subsets of patients with the so-called "minimal N2 disease" and some subgroups of T4 disease are widely accepted as potential candidates for surgical approaches [4–6]. Most stage IIIA/IIIB patients are not considered for surgery, and palliative systemic approaches consist of combinations of platinum-based chemotherapy and radiotherapy as standard of treatment [7].

The locally advanced stages IIIA and IIIB NSCLC have offered the best changes for possible therapeutic innovations and improvements. Several investigators have tested various treatment strategies in extended phase II and a small number of phase III trials [8–14]. Chemotherapy, alone or associated with radiotherapy, is used to downstage tumors and render them completely resectable. Cisplatin-based combination treatment was found to achieve response rates of 50% to 75% in localized unresectable disease and eradication of micrometastases was suggested. Preoperative radiotherapy resulted in sterilization of mediastinal nodes so that patients with initial unresectable disease underwent surgery. Whereas a possible survival improvement related to induction treatment before surgery was suggested, several studies highlighted postoperative risks with increase of morbidity and mortality [15–17]. Concurrent application of chemotherapy and radiation was considerably more toxic. Recent results of European Organisation for Research and Treatment of Cancer 08941 and the Intergroup study 0139 have shown, however, that the extent of surgery determines postoperative mortality and that only in a subgroup of patients with lobectomy was there a survival benefit [18,19].

The aim of the present contribution is to overview the literature and to evaluate the risks for medical and surgical complications of lung cancer surgery after induction chemotherapy or chemoradiotherapy in patients with locally advanced NSCLC. Obvious limitations of this report will be the complexity and heterogeneity of stage III disease in association with the difficult data collection of a large number of retrospective and small number of prospective randomized studies. The different definition of the time of postoperative mortality, as well the range of reported morbidity and mortality rates may reflect varying criteria for patient selection; differences in type and doses of induction treatment; and differences in the experiences of oncologists, radio-oncologists, and surgeons involved.

Morbidity and mortality after induction treatment

The results from retrospective studies analyzing postoperative mortality outside neoadjuvant

E-mail address: g.stamatis-ruhrlandklinik@t-online.de

1547-4127/08/$ - see front matter
doi:10.1016/j.thorsurg.2007.11.004

treatment showed mortality rates between 1.3% and 6.6% for overall mortality, 1.6% and 13.4% after pneumonectomy, and 0.6% and 4.0% after lobectomy [5,20–22]. Postoperative mortality after induction chemotherapy or chemoradiotherapy in phase II and randomized trials are summarized in Tables 1 and 2. However, these rates seem higher than what is reported after resection by monoinstitutional or multicenter databases suggesting an increased risk caused by the preoperative oncologic treatment, especially after chemoradiotherapy. Preoperative thoracic irradiation of more than 45 Gy proved to be a significant risk factor for postoperative complications in several but not in all studies. The association between higher-dose radiotherapy administered preoperatively and postoperative complications was first mentioned by Fowler and colleagues [15]. Thirteen patients were operated after a concurrent thoracic radiation with 60 Gy; excessive rates of morbidity (62%) and mortality (23%) were reported. After this report and the report of Deutsch and colleagues [31] with similar negative results, several large mono- or multi-institutional trials of induction chemoradiotherapy with a total radiation dose limited to 30 to 45 Gy followed by surgery were conducted [8–11]. Chemotherapy with concurrent radiotherapy limited to 45 Gy was proven to be safe and feasible in these trials and many investigators have used different ways to combine chemotherapy and radiotherapy protocols to optimize preoperative downsizing and downstaging [29,32–38] The mortality profile was associated with complications as bronchopleural fistula (BPF) and acute respiratory distress syndrome (ARDS), which occurred more frequently in patients after pneumonectomy [17,33,38]. The benefits of preoperative thoracic chemoradiotherapy resulted in increased pathological nodal downstaging, better disease-free survival, and the reduced risk for recurrence. These benefits must be weighed against the postoperative complications.

Table 1
Morbidity and mortality after induction chemotherapy in phase II and randomized studies

First author	Morbidity	Mortality
Martini [23]	—	5/114 (4.4%)
Rosell (1994) [13]	—	(7%)
Roth [12]	—	(0%)
Sugarbaker [24]	20/63 (31%)	2/63 (3.2%)
Doddoli [25]	35/69 (51%)	6/69 (9%)
Martin [17]	179/470 (38.1%)	18/470 (3.8%)
Siegenthaler [26]	34/76 (44.7%)	1/76 (1.3%)
Roberts [16]	16/34 (47.1%)	2/34 (5.8%)
Depierre [14]	—	(6.7%)
Perrot [27]	33/114 (28.9%)	2/114 (1.7%)
Pezzetta [28]		1/36 (3%)
EORTC 08941 (2005) [29]	—	6/149 (4%)
Brunelli [30]	18/70 (26%)	2/70 (2.9%)

Table 2
Morbidity and mortality after induction chemoradiotherapy in phase II and randomized studies

First author	Morbidity	Mortality
Fowler [15]	8/13 (62%)	3/13 (23%)
Deutsch [31]	3/16 (19%)	3/16 (19%)
Macchiarini [52]	6/23 (28%)	2/23 (8.6%)
Albain [8]	59/101 (58%)	8/101 (7.9%)
Rice [53]	11/36 (31%)	4/36 (11%)
Grunenwald [32]	7/29 (24%)	2/29 (7%)
DeCamp [54]	30/105 (31%)	7/105 (6.6%)
Stamatis [55]	180/392 (46%)	18/392 (4.6%)
Semik [33]	50/130 (38%)	8/130 (6.2%)
Intergroup 0139 [56]	—	10/202 (5%)
Pezzetta [28]	—	2/46 (4%)
Fujita [34]	54/124 (43.5%)	9/124 (7.3%)

In the last years, most investigations showed a clear learning curve in the morbidity and mortality analysis, and fewer adverse events usually appeared in the second half of the trials. Perioperative mortality has been reduced to approximately 1% to 2% for lobectomies and less than 6% for pneumonectomies, results comparable with series in which induction treatment included chemotherapy alone [27,30,39–42]. Learning effects also resulted in a small number of recent studies of safe surgical resections and reduced treatment-related mortality even when radiation doses of 58 to 61 Gy were used [43–46].

Age and gender

A number of quoted studies demonstrated that postoperative mortality was not significantly higher among older patients. However, the study populations were heterogeneous due to the inclusion of patients between 60 and 75 years so that the described results are statistically not comparable and the inclusion criteria for elderly patients requiring pneumonectomy was not well documented. Bernard and colleagues [20] found that mortality was higher in the population older than 70 without significant difference. In our study, univariate analysis demonstrated that higher age (>70 years) and lower performance status (Karnofsky index <80%) adversely affected the incidence of mortality [47]. Recent reports by Brouchet and colleagues [48] and Cerfolio and colleagues [49] confirm the higher risk for developing major morbidity in elderly patients if they underwent neoadjuvant treatment before resection. Harpole and colleagues [50] also pointed out that advanced age, right-side surgical procedures, and low FEV1 (forced expiratory volume in 1 second) were predictive of operative deaths and pulmonary complications in patients with pneumonectomy. Wada and colleagues [21] reported that in Japan, the low 30-day mortality rate of 3.2% is associated with a low proportion of pneumonectomies (8.3% of all resections), suggesting that elderly patients and patients with comorbidity possibly undergo less extensive procedures or receive nonsurgical treatments.

There are no differences in mortality between men and women in the most quoted studies. But recent reports showed than women respond better to neoadjuvant chemotherapy in stage IIIA disease with significantly better survival than men [51]. Brouchet and colleagues analyzed data of 555 patients who received induction chemotherapy between 2002 and 2004; using a multivariate analysis they found a significant correlation between morbidity and age (older than 65 years), sex (male), comorbidities (two or more), and type of operation (pneumonectomy/bilobectomy) [49]. In 193 consecutive pneumonectomy patients Licker and colleagues [22] pointed out that perioperative mortality was related mainly to hemorrhage, pneumonia, and multiple organ failure and occurred more frequently among the elderly men and patients with ASA classes 3 or 4.

Lung function and complications

Most patients who require pulmonary resection for lung cancer are smokers and often present with chronic obstructive and/or cardiopulmonary disease, so that pulmonary and cardiovascular complications (Table 3) are the most frequent, accounting for more than 85% of all complications [17,19,20]. Cardiac and pulmonary events occurring in the absence of concomitant surgical complications were shown to be an independent predictor of morbidity and mortality [25]. Even if smokers and patients with chronic obstructive pulmonary disease (COPD) participated in an intensive training and inhalative treatment with bronchodilators before surgery, complications such as pneumonia and atelectasis requiring bronchoscopy were observed. The rate of pneumonia varies in the literature from 3% to 19% (see Table 3), probably explained by the different criteria used to define postoperative pneumonia. We observed 19 cases of postoperative pneumonia, 4 of them with fatal outcome. Univariate and multivariate analysis identified lower performance status and higher age to be significant risk factors [55].Comparable results are published by others [17,25]. Prevention has been attributed to better preservation of the functional residual volume, efficient mucociliary clearance, and early function of diaphragm muscles. Early extubation, aggressive pulmonary toilet with bedside bronchoscopy, and efficient analgesia were recommended (Burfeind). Azad and colleagues [57] and Peeters-Asdourian and colleagues [58] demonstrated the benefit in patients with epidural analgesia and postoperative pain control. Variables measured bronchial obstruction as vital capacity (VC), forced vital capacity (FVC), and FEV1; also,

Table 3
Medical complications after induction treatment

First author	ARDS	Pneumonia	Atelectasis	Arrhythmia
Fowler [15]	6/13 (46%)	—	—	—
Martin [17]	19/470 (4%)	57/470 (12.1%)	39/470 (8.3%)	58 (12.3%)
Doddoli [25]	—	13/69 (19%)	5/69 (16%)	4/69 (5.7%)
Siegenthaler [26]	2/76 (2.6%)	8/76 (10.5%)	—	—
DeCamp [54]	3/98 (3%)	3/98 (3%)	—	18/98 (18%)
Stamatis [55]	7/392 (1.8%)	19/392 (4.8%)	17/392 (4.5%)	41/392 (10.6%)
Van Schil [29]	4/149 (2.7%)	9/!49 (6%)	4/149 (2.7%)	13/149 (8.7%)
Perrot [27]	3/114 (2.6%)	7/114 (6.1%)	—	5/114 (4.4%)
Pezzetta [28]	8/82 (9.7%)	4/82 (4.9%)	—	—

Abbreviation: ARDS, acute respiratory distress syndrome.

variables for gas exchange as diffusion capacity of the lung to carbon monoxide (DLCO) and oxygen saturation (SaO2) are analyzed in a number of retrospective reports [16,17,24,30,59–63]. In clinical practice, the postoperative predicted FEV1 and DLCO derived from a quantitative ventilation-perfusion scan and the preoperative pulmonary function tests are considered potential predictors of pulmonary complications. Martin and colleagues [17] highlighted that FEV1 (percent predicted) significantly predicts morbidity, DLCO (percent predicted) approaches significance as a predictor by univariate analysis, and that FEV1 is linearly correlated with DLCO. Leo and colleagues [59] and Takeda and colleagues [61] recommended DLCO studies before and after induction therapy because the decrease in DLCO is thought to reflect a limited gas exchange reserved due to potential toxicity of chemotherapy or chemoradiotherapy. Harpole and colleagues [64], Ferguson and colleagues [65], and Wang and colleagues [66] have extensively evaluated the postoperative risks after lung resection and have demonstrated that decreased DLCO is an accurate predictor of postoperative complications. Within the confines of all these retrospective studies, the thresholds that have been chosen to correspond to the lowest normal limits were different and it has not been possible to define an absolute cutoff point for FEV1 and DLCO in which most complications became unavoidable. Similar limitations were described by Kohman and colleagues [67], who evaluated 37 preoperative and 12 postoperative risk factors and found that all these factors together accounted for only 40% of perioperative morbidity. They concluded that the remainder of the risk of death must be attributed either to factors not considered or to purely randomized factors.

Respiratory failure and acute respiratory distress syndrome

The causes of postoperative pulmonary infiltrates still remain speculative. In some studies the incidence of postoperative ARDS was higher after neoadjuvant radiochemotherapy than after chemotherapy alone and was mainly observed after pneumonectomy but seldom after lobectomy [15,20,21,28,29,32,68]. Postpneumonectomy pulmonary edema has been described, usually occurring within the first 12 to 24 hours and different mechanisms such as lymphatic disruption, increased capillary pressure, and alveolar capillary injury are postulated. Increased perioperative fluid and crystalloid resuscitation as a cause of volume overload of the right ventricle and pulmonary circulation has been reported in the genesis of pulmonary edema [20,64]. Fowler and colleagues [15] found that respiratory complications are associated with the high intraoperative inspired oxygen tensions in patients with pulmonary limitations. Macchiarini and colleagues [52] and Martini and colleagues [23] estimated that this edema was primarily related to the pulmonary toxicity of mitomycin. The pneumotoxic effect of the mytomycin is probably increased by a preoperative 100% O2 delivery and combined radiotherapy doses of more than 45 Gy. Other factors such as the interruption of lymphatic drainage of the remaining lung due to extensive lymph node dissection, explain why this edema is more frequent after right pneumonectomy associated with a more radical nodal resection than on the left side. The only reports that found no increased incidence in these complications in 19 consecutive patients who all received radiation of more than 59 Gy was published by Sonnett and colleagues [43] and by Daly and colleagues [44]. There are, however, a variety of options that can be used to decrease the likelihood of ARDS and pulmonary edema–related deaths after induction treatment. These include intraoperative and postoperative fluid restriction; the avoidance of high oxygen delivery intraoperatively, which can act in synergy with drugs resulting in lung damage; the avoidance of aggressive lymph node dissection in the contralateral mediastinum with interruption of the lymphatic drainage of the remaining lung; the use of bronchovascular sleeve resections instead of pneumonectomy if it is technically possible; and the use of prophylactic steroids over a short period of time [69]. To reduce tissue edema, prednisolone 1 mg/kg body weight was given by our group for a period of 3 days starting in the operating theater [47]. That is an anecdotally supported practice also reported by different authors [15,54,69].

Cardiovascular complications

Preexisting cardiovascular disease is one of the strongest predictors of morbidity and mortality. The presence of concomitant cardiovascular disease was associated with increased mortality in patients after pneumonectomy [20,22,64].

Arrhythmias occurred in 4% to 18% (see Table 3) of the patients, and coronary artery disease could be preoperatively identified as a risk factor. The incidence of arrhythmias could also be explained by appropriate perioperative control of pain, hypovolemia, anemia, and hypercoagulation [22]. However, atrial fibrillation was observed in patients with coexisting pneumonia and respiratory failure [20]. Advanced age (>70 years) and extended resections (pneumonectomy), respectively, in advanced stages (III and IV) were predictive of cardiac arrhythmias in two reports [22,47]. In our series, arrhythmias occurred in 13% of all patients and in 27% of those after pneumonectomy. Because of known myocardial toxicity of chemotherapeutics, drugs, and radiotherapy, all patients were investigated before surgery with echocardiography and, in case of abnormal findings, with stress electrocardiogram. Such a selective screening approach is helpful in identifying patients who require more intensive perioperative care and are eligible for resection, and also to exclude those with poor ventricular function.

Thromboembolic complications

The incidence of reported postoperative pulmonary thromboembolic episodes is low, the reported range is from 0% to1.7% [20,29,47]. Pulmonary thromboembolism after lung resection is associated with high mortality and is a frequent cause of acute fatal outcome after pneumonectomy. We observed pulmonary thromboembolism in about 4% of patients without any clinical symptoms or functional limitations or subsegmental or segmental failures in the perfusion scan done after induction chemoradiotherapy and before surgery. For this group, prophylactic anticoagulation with low molecular weight heparin was used, started 1 week before pulmonary resection. Doddoli and colleagues [68] postulated than the sudden deaths with unknown origin in otherwise healthy discharged patients after induction treatment and pneumonectomy might have been caused by pulmonary embolism. He recommended the use of vitamin K antagonist in the long run.

Hemorrhage and blood transfusion

Pulmonary and cardiac events are often associated with allogeneic blood transfusions. Blood requirements depend on preoperative hemoglobin levels; it might be anticipated that induction chemotherapy and anemia increase these needs. This fact is of clinical relevance because data on transfusion therapy have not always been favorable, particularly in the areas of postoperative infection, systemic inflammatory response, and multiple organ failure [68]. Bernard and colleagues [20] reported that low serum hemoglobin levels were associated with increased mortality in patients with pneumonectomy. Also, Harpole and colleagues [64] observed a correlation between a low hematocrit value and the onset of atrial fibrillation after pneumonectomy. In our series, blood transfusion did not affected postoperative mortality [55]. Also, in the published study by Perrot and colleagues [27], postoperative morbidity was not higher among patients with hemoglobin lower than 12 g/dL. Prevention of intraoperative complications is the key to reducing perioperative mortality. In several series, hemorrhage was responsible for complicated outcomes, especially in patients with extended tumors or/and hilar irradiation. In the presence of extensive perihilar adhesions, freeing of the pulmonary artery and its branches in the major fissure can be quite difficult, even for an experienced thoracic surgeon, necessitating intrapericardial, retrograde, or posterior dissection [29]. Reintervention because of postoperative bleeding was reported in 0.8% to 2.6% of the cases. We tend to reoperate the patients as early as possible so that further complications can be reduced.

Air leakage and prolonged hospital stay

Despite meticulous preparation of interlobar fissure and hilar structures, the incidence of air leakage after lobectomy or bilobectomy (Table 4) was higher compared with historical collectives without induction, probably related to adhesiolysis or tissue damage induced by lung radiation. Also, changes in the structure of interlobar and hilar nodes as a result of chemotherapy or chemoradiotherapy resulted in lung parenchyma injury during their removal with prolonged postoperative air leakage. The reported average hospital stay of between 12 and 22 days confirms the different outcome to collectives without induction treatment [17,25,28,32,38,55].

The risk of right-side pneumonectomy and bronchopleural fistula

Advances in perioperative management have improved surgical outcome for pulmonary resection, but pneumonectomy continues to be

Table 4
Surgical complications after induction treatment

First author	BPF	Empyema	Bleeding	Prolonged air leakage
Fowler [15]	3/13 (23%)	—	—	1/6 (16.6%)
Martin [17]	8/470 (1.7%)	6/470 (1.3%)	39/470 (8.3%)	45/315 (14.2%)
Doddoli [25]	5/69 (7.2%)	—	1/69 (16%)	5/32 (16%)
DeCamp [54]	3/98 (3%)	—	1/98 (1%)	13/98 (3%)
Stamatis [55]	16/392 (3.2%)	6/392 (1.6%)	10/392 (2.5%)	34/244 (13.9%)
Van Schil [29]	5/149 (3.4%)	11/149 (7.4%)	4/149 (2.7%)	12/149 (8%)
Perrot [27]	0/114 (0%)	—	5/114 (4.4%)	4/114 (3.5%)
Pezzetta [28]	4/82 (4.9%)	—	—	—

Abbreviation: BPF, bronchopleural fistula.

associated with the highest complication and mortality rate of all elective thoracic surgery [20,22,70]. It has been suggested that the mortality of a right pneumonectomy is higher than on the left side. Before the introduction of multimodality treatments, a few reports compared outcomes after right and left pneumonectomies. Wahi and colleagues [71] first reported that right pneumonectomy was associated with higher mortality than the left (12% versus 1%). Au and colleagues [72] found significantly higher mortality after right pneumonectomy in elderly patients (37% versus 6%). A milestone paper in the recent literature regarding the risks of pneumonectomy after induction is the report of Martin and colleagues [17]. The authors conclude that surgery after induction treatment is associated with an acceptable overall morbidity and mortality but they alerted that right pneumonectomy is associated with a mortality rate of 23.9% at 3 months, whereas there was no mortality following left pneumonectomy. The frightening 90-day mortality could partially be explained by the use of mitomycin-based chemotherapies. It remains surprising that there was no mortality after left pneumonectomy. Several other authors reported an adverse effect [20,28,38,68]. Initial results of the North American Intergroup Trial 0139 showed in the induction therapy surgery arm a mortality of 22% (5/23) after simple and 29% (9/31) after complex pneumonectomy, but only 1% (1/98) after lobectomy [56]. It was postulated that the increased risk of right pneumonectomy may be related to the increased load on the right ventricle of the entire cardiac output going through the smaller left lung, resulting in increased pulmonary artery pressures, pulmonary hypertension, and right ventricular failure [73].

The high mortality rates also might be explained by a magnification of the higher risk of BPF and respiratory failure of the right-sided procedures [74,75]. The overall incidence of BPF reported in most recent series varies between 0% and 9% (Table 5). The bronchial stump must be managed with meticulous care, avoiding devascularization and excessive length. More extensive resection and aggressive lymphadenectomy with removal of the surrounding fat and devitalization of peribronchial tissue in addition to a high dose of radiotherapy of more than 45 to 50 Gy were supposed as important factors favoring bronchial fistulas. The increased frequency of BPF on the right side could be explained by the anatomic difference of more exposure in the pleural space and less naturally buttressed by mediastinal structures. Darling and colleagues [73] highlighted that attention must be directed to ensuring that there is no tension on the bronchial closure. The cartilaginous ring at the origin of the right main bronchus

Table 5
Rates of mortality and bronchopleural fistula after induction treatment and pneumonectomy

First author	No. of pneumonectomies	Mortality (%)	BPF (%)
Fowler [15]	7	43	14
Martin [17]	97	23.9	1.7
Siegenthaler [26]	8	0	0
Stamatis [55]	133	7.1	9
Doddoli [68]	100	12	6
Van Schil [29]	69	7.2	7.2
Perrot [27]	27	1.8	0
Port [80]	15	6.6	—
Pezzetta [28]	34	2.9	—
Intergroup [56]	54	25	—
Mansour [39]	60	6.7	1.7

Abbreviation: BPF, bronchopleural fistula.

has a tendency to keep the bronchus open. A portion of this ring should be resected to allow the bronchus to be closed without tension.

The bronchial suture was preferentially made with a stapling device by the majority of surgeons. The preference of all authors is to reinforce the bronchial stump with viable tissue, especially on the right side. The analysis of our data identified that the bronchial stump–covering technique is a highly effective procedure to prevent BPF with statistical significance [47]. The use of pericardium, the azygos vein, intercostals muscle or other thoracic skeletal muscles, diaphragm, mediastinal fat/thymus flap, and omental flap has been reported by different authors [32,39,55,73,76]. We routinely covered the bronchial stump following right-sided pneumonectomy with a pericardial/thymic fat pad placed below the superior vena cava. The blood supply from the pericardiophrenic artery is excellent and the tissue volume usually sufficient. There are only a few series that showed that induction therapy did not increase the operative risks in patients with pneumonectomy [26,27,39]. In this group of patients, only chemotherapy was used before surgery and the limited number of complications were explained by the selection of the patients and the specialization of the units, with a high volume of thoracotomies performed exclusively by thoracic surgeons.

As alternative procedures to pneumonectomy, bronchoplastic and angioplastic techniques with preservation of lung parenchyma were recommended [28,70,77,78]. Sleeve lobectomy can be accomplished with a much lower operative mortality rate than pneumonectomy (1.3% versus 5.3%). If complete resection can be performed by bronchoplastic techniques, these patients will enjoy longer survival and better local control than will pneumonectomy patients [70]. After induction treatment, lobectomy associated with bronchial and/or vascular reconstruction is technically demanding, and complex bronchovascular reconstructions are even more so. The procedure is generally more difficult than in other settings because of a variable degree of fibrosis [28,29,55,74,77]. This fibrosis renders surgical dissection more tedious at the sites of initial involvement of different lymph nodal stations because the hilar and mediastinal regions are frequently involved. All resectioned margins, especially the bronchial sleeve, have to be checked by intraoperative frozen section and sleeve resection should be extended to reach healthy tissue [77]. Of the potential for complications associated with bronchoplastic resections after induction therapy, anastomotic complications are the most important. Preoperative chemoradiotherapy adversely affects mucosal blood flow and healing [79], prompting recommendations to protect the anastomosis with well-vascularized flaps and to separate it from the pulmonary artery.

Nevertheless, reports about increased risks of right pneumonectomy triggered some consideration of pneumonectomy as a routine procedure, the danger being that operable patients could be denied for surgery. Does this mean that one should stop doing right pneumonectomy? Obviously, the answer is no because bronchial or and vascular sleeve resections is not applicable in all patients and for some individuals it is the only available option if one is to completely resect the cancer. Pneumonectomy is an operation that thoracic surgeons should not fear but rather should be done with confidence when it is needed.

Summary

Pulmonary resection for locally advanced NSCLC after induction chemotherapy or chemoradiotherapy can generally be performed with acceptable morbidity and mortality. Data from several phase II and a few randomized trials showed that patients should be carefully selected for surgery especially with respect to their age, performance status, and pulmonary and cardiovascular function tests. The presence of cardiovascular disease should be actively investigated and preexisting arrhythmias appropriately managed. Similarly, respiratory status should be evaluated and any reversible condition, such bronchial obstruction, infection, pulmonary embolism, and smoking, should be addressed. Surgical resection is technically more demanding; intraoperative blood loss should be minimized. Several studies demonstrated that pneumonectomy especially on the right side is associated with a significantly increased risk of postoperative morbidity and mortality especially in patients after induction chemoradiotherapy. Therefore, pneumonectomy should be performed very selectively and only when alternative procedures such as bronchial or vascular sleeve resection or both are technically not possible. Long-term follow-up reports of bimodality protocols without surgery versus bimodality followed by surgical resection are awaited. These results will help to define standards of care and the role of surgery for patients with NSCLC stage III disease. Future decision-making will have to take into account treatment morbidity and mortality and parameters of organ-sparing surgery following induction, probably best represented by rates of pneumonectomy or rates of lobectomy in different patient groups.

References

[1] Levi F, Lucchini F, Negri E, et al. Cancer mortality in Europe 1995–1999, and an overview of trends since 1960. Int J Cancer 2004;1105:155–69.

[2] Jemal A, Tiwari RC, Murray T, et al. Cancer statistics, 2004. CA Cancer J Clin 2004;54(1):8–29.

[3] Ginsberg RJ, Vokes EE, Raben A. Non-small cell lung cancer. In: De Vita VT Jr, Hellmann S, Rosenberg SA, editors. Cancer: principles and practice of oncology. 5th edition. Philadelphia: Lippincott; 1997. p. 858–911.

[4] Fabrice A, Grunenwald D, Pignon JP, et al. Survival of patients with resected N2 non small cell lung cancer (NSCLC): heterogeneity of prognosis and evidence for a subclassification (abstract). Proc Am Soc Clin Oncol 1999;18:1802.

[5] Van Raemdonck DE, Schneider A, GinsbergRJ. Surgical treatment for higher stage non-small cell lung cancer. Ann Thorac Surg 1992;54:999–1013.

[6] Mathisen DJ, Grillo HC. Carinal resection for bronchogenic carcinoma. J Thorac Cardiovasc Surg 1988;102:16–23.

[7] Johnson DH, Turrisi AT, Pass HJ. Combined modality treatment for locally advanced non-small cell lung cancer. In: Pass HJ, Mitchell J, Johnson DH, Turrisi AT, editors. Lung cancer: principles and practice. Philadelphia: Lippincott; 1996. p. 863–73.

[8] Albain KS, Rush V, Crowley J, et al. Concurrent cisplatin/etoposide plus chest radiotherapy followed by surgery for stages IIIA (N2) and IIIB non-small cell lung cancer: major mature results of Southwest Oncology Group phase II study 8805. J Clin Oncol 1995;13:1880–92.

[9] Choi N, Carey R, Daly W, et al. Potential impact on survival of improved tumor downstaging and resection rate by preoperative twice-daily radiation and concurrent chemotherapy in stage IIIA non-small cell lung cancer. J Clin Oncol 1997;15:712–22.

[10] Eberhardt W, Wilke H, Stamatis G, et al. Preoperative chemotherapy followed by concurrent chemoradiation therapy based on hyperfractionated accelerated radiotherapy and definitive surgery in locally advanced non-small cell lung cancer: mature results of a phase II trial. J Clin Oncol 1998;16:622–34.

[11] Thomas M, Rübe C, Semik M, et al. Chemotherapy and subsequent twice-daily chemoradiation before surgery in stage III non-small cell lung cancer: impact of tumor regression on survival. J Clin Oncol 1999;17:1185–93.

[12] Roth JA, Fossela FV, Komaki R, et al. A randomised trial comparing preoperative chemotherapy and surgery with surgery alone in resectable stage IIIA non-small cell lung cancer. J Natl Cancer Inst 1994;86:673–80.

[13] Rossell R, Gomez-Codina J, Camps C, et al. A randomized trial comparing preoperative chemotherapy plus surgery with surgery alone in patients with non-small cell lung cancer. N Engl J Med 1994;330:153–8.

[14] Depierre A, Milleron B, Moro-Sibilot D, et al. Preoperative chemotherapy followed by surgery compared with primary surgery in resectable stage I (except T1N0), II and IIIA non-small cell lung cancer. J Clin Oncol 2002;20:247–53.

[15] Fowler WC, Langer CJ, Curran WJ, et al. Postoperative complications after combined neoadjuvant treatment of lung cancer. Ann Thorac Surg 1993; 55:986–9.

[16] Roberts JR, Eustis C, Devore R, et al. Induction chemotherapy increases perioperative complications in patients undergoing resection for non-small cell lung cancer. Ann Thorac Surg 2001;72:885–8.

[17] Martin J, Ginsberg RJ, Abolhoda A, et al. Morbidity and mortality after neoadjuvant therapy for lung cancer: The risks of right pneumonectomy. Ann Thorac Surg 2001;72:1149–54.

[18] Albain KS, Scott CB, Rusch VW, et al. Phase III study of concurrent chemotherapy and full course radiotherapy (CT/RT) versus CT/RT induction followed by surgical resection for stage IIIA(N2) non-small cell lung cancer (NSCLC): first outcome analysis of North American Intergroup trial 0139 (RTOG 93–09). Lung Cancer 2003;41(Suppl 2):S4.

[19] Van Meerbeeck JP, van Schil PE, Seuan S, et al. Randomized controlled trial of resection versus radiotherapy after induction chemotherapy in stage IIIA N2 non-small cell lung cancer. J Natl Cancer Inst 2007;99:442–50.

[20] Bernard A, Deschamps C, Allen MS, et al. Peumonectomy for malignant disease: factors affecting early morbidity and mortality. J Thorac Cardiovasc Surg 2001;121:1076–82.

[21] Wada H, Nakamura T, Nakamoto K, et al. Thirty-day operative mortality for thoracotomy in lung cancer. Thorac Cardiovasc Surg 1998;115:70–3.

[22] Licker M, Spiliopoulos A, Frey JG, et al. Risk factors for early mortality and major complications following pneumonectomy for non-small cell carcinoma of the lung. Chest 2002;121:1890–7.

[23] Martini N, Kris MG, Flehinger BJ, et al. Preoperative chemotherapy for stage IIIA (N2): the Sloan-Kattering experience with 136 patients. Ann Thorac Surg 1993;55:1365–74.

[24] Sugarbaker DJ, Herndorn J, Kohman LJ, et al. Results of cancer and leukaemia group B protocol 8935: a multiinstitutional phase II trimodality trial

for stage IIIA (N2) non-small cell lung cancer. J Thorac Cardiovasc Surg 1995;109:473–85.
[25] Doddoli C, Thomas P, Thirion X, et al. Postoperative complications in relation with induction therapy for lung cancer. Eur J Cardiothorac Surg 2001;20:385–90.
[26] Siegenthaler MP, Pisters KM, Merriman KW, et al. Preoperative chemotherapy for lung cancer does not increase surgical morbidity. Ann Thorac Surg 2001;71:1105–12.
[27] Perrot E, Guibert B, Mulsant P, et al. Preoperative chemotherapy does not increase complications after non-small cell lung cancer resection. Ann Thorac Surg 2005;80:423–7.
[28] Pezzetta E, Stupp R, Zouhair A, et al. Comparison of neoadjuvant cisplatin-based chemotherapy versus chemoradiotherapy followed by resection for stage III(N2) NSCLC. Eur J Cardiothorac Surg 2005;27:1092–8.
[29] Van Schil P, van Meerbeeck J, Kramer G, et al. Morbidity and mortality in surgery arm of EORTC 08941 trial. Eur Respir J 2005;26:192–7.
[30] Brunelli A, Xiumé F, Refai MA, et al. Gemcitabine-cisplatin chemotherapy before lung resection: a case-matched analysis of early outcome. Ann Thorac Surg 2006;81:1963–8.
[31] Deutsch M, Crawford J, Leopold K, et al. Phase II study of neoadjuvant chemotherapy and radiation therapy with thoracotomy in the treatment of clinically staged IIIA non-small cell lung cancer. Cancer 1994;74:1243–52.
[32] Grunenwald DH, André F, Le Péchoux C, et al. Benefit of surgery after chemoradiortherapy in stage IIIB (T4 and/or N3) non-small cell lung cancer. J Thorac Cardiovasc Surg 2001;122:796–802.
[33] Semik M, Riesenbeck D, Linder A, et al. Preoperative chemotherapy with and without additional radiochemotherapy: benefit and risk for surgery of stage III non-small cell lung cancer. Eur J Cardiothorac Surg 2004;26:1205–10.
[34] Fujita S, Katakami N, Takahashi Y, et al. Postoperative complications after induction chemoradiotherapy in patients with non small cell lung cancer. Eur J Cardiothorac Surg 2006;29:896–901.
[35] Machtay M, Lee JH, Stevenson JP, et al. Two commonly used neoadjuvant chemoradiotherapy regimens for locally advanced stage III non-small cell lung carcinoma: long term results and associations with pathologic response. J Thorac Cardiovasc Surg 2004;127:108–13.
[36] Gauler T, Eberhardt W, Le Pechoux C, et al. Multicenter German/French phase II trial of induction CTX followed by concurrent CTX/RTX+/−surgery in locally for advanced inoperable non-small cell lung cancer stages IIIA (N2) and IIIB-mature results of a novel induction CTX regimen. J Cancer Res Clin Oncol 2004;130:S72.
[37] Friedel G, Budach W, Sprengler W, et al. Phase II trial on neo-adjuvant chemoradiation with paclitaxel/carboplatin in stage III NSCLC. J Cancer Res Clin Oncol 2004;130:S72.
[38] Venouta F, Anile M, Diso D, et al. Operative complications and early mortality after induction therapy for lung cancer. Eur J Cardiothorac Surg 2007;31:714–8.
[39] Mansour Z, Kochetkova EA, Ducrocq X, et al. Induction chemotherapy does not increase the operative risk of pneumonectomy. Eur J Cardiothorac Surg 2007;31:181–5.
[40] Takeda S, Maeda H, Okada T, et al. Results of pulmonary resection following neoadjuvant therapy for locally advanced (IIIA-IIIB) lung cancer. Eur J Cardiothoracic Surg 2006;30:184–9.
[41] Gilligan D, Nicolson M, Smith I, et al. Preoperative chemotherapy in patients with resectable non-small cell lung cancer: results of the MRC LU22/NVALT 2/EORTC 08012 multicentre randomised trial and update of systematic review. Lancet 2007;369:1929–37.
[42] Yokomise H, Gotoh M, Okamoto T, et al. Induction chemoradiotherapy (carboplatin-taxane and concurrent 50-Gy radiation) for bulky cN2, N3 non-small cell lung cancer. J Thorac Cardiovasc Surg 2007;133:1179–85.
[43] Sonnett JR, Krasna MJ, Suntharalingam M, et al. Safe pulmonary resection after chemotherapy and high-dose thoracic radiation. Ann Thorac Surg 1999;68:316–20.
[44] Daly BDT, Fernando HC, Ketchedjian A, et al. Pneumonectomy after high-dose radiation and concurrent chemotherapy for nonsmall cell lung cancer. Ann Thorac Surg 2006;82:227–31.
[45] Cerfolio RJ, Bryant AS, Spencer Sa, et al. Pulmonary resection after high-dose and low-dose chest irradiation. Ann Thorac Surg 2005;80:1224–30.
[46] Shaikh AY, Haraf DJ, Salama JK, et al. Chemotherapy and high dose radiotherapy followed by resection in locally advanced nonsmall cell lung cancer. Am J Clin Oncol 2007;30:258–63.
[47] Stamatis G, Djuric D, Eberhardt W, et al. Postoperative morbidity and mortality after induction chemotherapy for locally advanced lung cancer: an analysis of 350 operated patients. Eur J Cardiothorac Surg 2002;22:292–7.
[48] Brouchet L, Bauvin E, Marcheix B, et al. Impact of induction treatment on postoperative complications in the treatment of non-small cell lung cancer. J Thorac Oncol 2007;2:626–31.
[49] Cerfolio RJ, Bryant AS. Survival and outcomes of pulmonary resection for non-small cell lung cancer in the elderly: a nested case-control study. Ann Thorac Surg 2006;82:424–9.
[50] Harpole DH, Liptay MJ, DeCamp MM, et al. Prospective analysis of pneumonectomy: risk factors fro major morbidity and cardiac dysrhythmias. Ann Thorac Surg 1996;61:977–82.
[51] Cerfolio RJ, Bryant AS, Scott E, et al. Women with pathologic stage I, II, and III non-small cell lung

cancer have better survival than men. Chest 2006; 130:1796–802.
[52] Macchiarini P, Chapelier AR, Monet I, et al. Extended operations after induction stage IIIB (T4) non-small cell lung cancer. Ann Thorac Surg 1994; 57:966–73.
[53] Rice TW, Adelstein DJ, Koka A, et al. Accelerated induction therapy and resection for poor prognosis Stage III non-small cell lung cancer. Ann Thorac Surg 1995;60:586–92.
[54] DeCamp MM, Rice TW, Adelstein DJ, et al. Value of accelerated multimodality therapy in stage IIIA and IIIB non-small cell lung cancer. J Thorac Cardiovasc Surg 2003;121:17–27.
[55] Stamatis G, Eberhardt W, Pöttgen C. Surgery after multimodality treatment for non-small cell lung cancer. Lung Cancer 2004;45(Suppl 2):107–12.
[56] Albain KS, Swann RS, Rusch VR, et al. Phase III study of concurrent chemotherapy and radiotherapy(CT/RT) vs. CT/RT followed by surgical resection for stage IIIA(N2) non-small cell lung cancer (NSCL): outcomes update of North American Intergroup 0139 (RTOG 9309). ASCO 2005 Abstract No: 7014.
[57] Azad SC, Groh J, Beyer A, et al. Continuous peridural analgesia vs. patient-controlled intravenous analgesia for pain therapy after thoracotomy. Anaesthesist 2000;49:9–17.
[58] Peeters-Asdourian G, Gupta S. Choices in pain management following thoracotomy. Chest 1999; 115(Suppl):1228–48.
[59] Leo F, Solli P, Spaggiari, et al. Respiratory function changes after chemotherapy: an additional risk factor for postoperative respiratory complications. Ann Thorac Surg 2004;77:260–5.
[60] Brunelli A, Refai M, Salati M, et al. Predicted versus observed FEV1 and DLCO after major lung resection: a prospective evaluation at different postoperative periods. Ann Thorac Surg 2007;83:1134–9.
[61] Takeda S, Funakoshi Y, Kadota Y, et al. Fall in diffusing capacity associated with induction therapy for lung cancer: a preditor of postoperative complications? Ann Thorac Surg 2006;82:232–6.
[62] Abou-Jawde RM, Mekhail T, Adelstein DJ, et al. Impact of induction chemoradiotherapy on pulmonary function and postoperative acute respiratory complications in esophageal cancer. Chest 2005; 128:250–5.
[63] Videtic GM, Stitt LW, Ash RB, et al. Impaired diffusion capacity predicts for decreased treatment tolerance and survival in limited stage small cell lung cancer treated with concurrent chemoradiation. Lung Cancer 2004;43:159–66.
[64] Harpole DH, DeCamp MM, Daley J, et al. Prognostic models of thirty-day mortality and morbidity after major pulmonary resection. J Thorac Cardiovasc Surg 1999;117:969–79.
[65] Ferguson MK, Reeder LB, Mick R. Optimizing selection of patients for major lung resection. J Thorac Cardiovasc Surg 1996;61:977–82.
[66] Wang J, Olak J, Ultmann RE, et al. Assessment of pulmonary complications after lung resection. Ann Thorac Surg 1999;67:1444–7.
[67] Kohman LJ, Meyer JA, Ikins PM, et al. Random versus predictable risks of mortality after thoracotomy for lung cancer. J Thorac Cardiovasc Surg 1986;91:551–4.
[68] Doddoli C, Barlesi F, Trousse D, et al. One hundred consecutive pneumonectomies after induction therapy for non-small cell lung cancer: An uncertain balance between risks and benefits. J Thorac Cardiovasc Surg 2005;130:416–25.
[69] Deslauriers J. Invited commentary. Ann Thorac Surg 2001;72:1154.
[70] Deslauriers J, Grégoire J, Jacques LF, et al. Sleeve lobectomy vs pneumonectomy for lung cancer: a comparative analysis of survival and sites of recurrences. Ann Thorac Surg 2004;77:1152–6.
[71] Wahi R, Mc Murtrey MJ, De Caro LF, et al. Determinants of perioperative morbidity and mortality after pneumonectomy. Ann Thorac Surg 1989;48: 33–7.
[72] Au J, elOakley R, Cameron EW. Pneumonectomy for bronchogenic carcinoma in the elderly. Eur J Cardiovasc Surg 1994;8:247–50.
[73] Darling GE, Abdurahman A, Yi QL, et al. Risk of a right pneumonectomy: role of bronchopleural fistula. Ann Thorac Surg 2005;79:433–7.
[74] Liptay MJ, Frey WA. Complications from induction regimens for thoracic malignancies. Perioperative considerations. Chest Surg Clin N Am 1999;9: 79–95.
[75] Deschamps C, Bernard A, Nichols FC, et al. Empyema and bronchopleural fistula after pneumonectomy: factors affecting incidence. Ann Thorac Surg 2001;72:243–8.
[76] Levashev YN, Akopov AL, Mosin IV. The possibilities of greater omentum usage in thoracic surgery. Eur J Cardiothorac Surg 1999;15:465–8.
[77] Rendina AE, Venuta F, De Giacomo T, et al. Safety and efficacy of bronchovascular reconstruction after induction chemotherapy for lung cancer. J Thorac Cardiovasc Surg 1997;114:830–7.
[78] Burnfeind WR, D'Amico TA, Toloza EM, et al. Low morbidity and mortality for bronchoplastic procedures with and without induction treatment. Ann Thorac Surg 2005;80:418–22.
[79] Yamamoto R, Tada H, Kishi A, et al. Effect of preoperative chemotherapy and radiation therapy on human bronchial blood flow. J Thorac Cardiovasc Surg 2000;119:939–45.
[80] Port JL, Korst RJ, Lee PC, et al. Surgical resection for residual N2 disease after induction chemotherapy. Ann Thorac Surg 2005;79:1686–90.

ELSEVIER
SAUNDERS

Thorac Surg Clin 18 (2008) 81–91

THORACIC
SURGERY
CLINICS

Long-Term Quality of Life After Lung Resection

John Cannon, MBBS, MRCP, Thida Win, MD, MRCP*

Respiratory Medicine, Lister Hospital, Stevenage, SG1 4AB, UK

In 1949, Karnofsky and Burchenal [1] first introduced the concept of quality of life (QOL) as one of the indices to evaluate performance status in the treatment of chemotherapy for cancer patients. In 1976, Priestman and Baum [2] reported that postoperative psychologic disorders in patients with breast cancer had been improved with counseling. Since then psychiatrists and oncologists have investigated the social, mental, and behavioral problems of cancer patients. The term "QOL" has been widely referred to by physicians. One of the main issues for studying QOL in cancer patients was how to establish reliable measurement tools for QOL. Many proposals for measuring QOL of cancer patients have been reported [3–5].

The QOL has at least two implications in terms of definition [4]. The first is related to psychologic or ethical issues. These are issues related to living to some purpose in one's daily and social life or maintaining a good relationship with family and friends. The second is related to physical issues, such as physical function and working capability, which are affected by physical sensations like pain, sleep, appetite, and secretions. Schipper and coworkers [5] defined that QOL was composed of four elements: (1) working capability in one's daily life, (2) psychologic status, (3) ability to maintain human relations, and (4) degree of comfort or discomfort in physical sensation.

The long-term consequences of the curative treatment for non–small cell lung cancer (NSCLC) on pulmonary status, the frequency of respiratory symptoms, and the impact of these on the QOL of survivors have rarely been reported. Respiratory distress may negatively affect QOL even among the 14% of patients with NSCLC who are disease-free survivors [6]. Dyspnea and other respiratory symptoms have been reported to impact QOL negatively in those with chronic obstructive pulmonary disease and other chronic lung conditions [7–10] but little information is available about the impact on people with cancer [11]. One study [12] suggests that patients with NSCLC may actually have better QOL than those with severe chronic obstructive pulmonary disease. The perception of respiratory symptoms among long-term survivors of lung cancer may be affected by many variables. For instance aging, tobacco use, and comorbid conditions in particular may influence respiratory symptoms and level of pulmonary function [13,14]. About half of lung cancer patients have already stopped smoking at the time of diagnosis [15]; however tobacco-related effects on pulmonary function and respiratory symptoms can continue. Gender differences in respiratory symptoms among lung cancer patients have also been reported [16]. Most available reports of the pulmonary status and QOL of survivors of NSCLC only provide information over a relatively short-term period following surgery [17–22].

Health-related quality of life assessment

Quality of life questionnaires

There are several tools for quality of life assessment. Among these, EORTC QLQ-C30 and QLQ-LC13 are the most commonly used questionnaires [23–27]. The EORTC QLQ-C30 includes five functional scales (physical, role, emotional, social, and cognitive functioning); three symptom scales (fatigue, pain, and nausea-vomiting); a global health status and quality of life scale; and a number of single items assessing additional symptoms and perceived financial impact. The QLQ-LC13

* Corresponding author.
E-mail address: thida.win@nhs.net (T. Win).

1547-4127/08/$ - see front matter
doi:10.1016/j.thorsurg.2007.10.004

assesses lung cancer–specific symptoms, such as cough, hemoptysis, severity of shortness of breath, chest and body pain, and chemotherapy and radiotherapy side effects symptoms, such as sore mouth, dysphagia, peripheral neuropathy, and hair loss. All scales are reweighted to a scale of 0 to 100 according to the EORTC manual for the core questionnaire and the lung cancer module. A high score (60–100) represents a high-healthy level of functioning for a functional scale and a high global quality of life. A high score (60–100) for a symptom scale, however, represents a high level of symptomatology.

The EORTC QLQ-LC13 is a supplemental questionnaire module that was designed for use among patients receiving treatment with chemotherapy or radiotherapy. It contains 13 questions or items assessing lung cancer–associated symptoms (cough, hemoptysis, dyspnea, and site-specific pain); chemotherapy- or radiotherapy-related side effects (sore mouth, dysphagia, peripheral neuropathy, and alopecia); and pain medication. The dyspnea scale is aggregated into a four-item scale by including the single dyspnea item of the EORTC QLQ-C30 core questionnaire. Reliability and validity of the EORTC QLQ-LC13 module have been confirmed in international studies [28,29].

The Lung Cancer Symptom scale is also used in some studies [30,31]. The Hospital Anxiety Depression (HAD) scale [32], preoperative psychologic global well-being index [33], and the Medical Outcomes Study 36-item short form (SF-36) [27,32] were used to compare more general symptoms. The SF-36 instrument is designed to evaluate health-related QOL (HRQOL) in multiple groups of patients. It is composed of 36 items, grouped into eight scales, which include both physical and mental health, and assesses eight dimensions of QOL. The raw subscale scores are standardized and range from 0 to 100, where 0 represents the poorest state of health and 100 the best possible. Two summary scores are also calculated (the physical component summary scores and the mental component summary scores) to summarize the physical and mental state of health. The HAD scale is a brief self-administered rating scale designed to measure anxiety and depression in somatically ill individuals. The questionnaire contains 14 items for self-assessment on a scale of 0 to 3. Seven questions are related to anxiety and seven to depression, with a scale range of 0 to 21 for both variables. A score of eight or more on each subscale represents "possible" psychiatric morbidity and a score of 11 or more represents "definite" clinical anxiety or depression. The depression subscale has been constructed so that somatic items are largely excluded. Three lung-specific questions were used: patients were asked to rate the presence of pain in the chest, breathlessness, and cough on a scale of 1 to 4 during the last week. Patients also answered questions about their smoking history. For specific QOL assessment, Functional Assessment of Cancer Therapy—lung [34] was used.

Quality of life and respiratory symptoms in lung cancer patients

Symptom reports in lung cancer patients have primarily focused on advanced-stage disease, but most support the importance of symptom burden on QOL [22,35]. In a longer-term follow-up, two thirds of the survivors reported at least one respiratory symptom, with dyspnea and wheezing being the most common complaints. Combinations of symptoms, such as cough and phlegm, were also common and 11% of survivors described themselves as so breathless they could not leave the house [36]. Clinical QOL studies in unselected lung cancer patients reported pain in 86%, dyspnea in 70%, and anorexia in 68% [37].

The presence of respiratory symptoms contributed to perceptions relating to all dimensions of QOL, except mental health. Not unexpectedly, the presence of dyspnea was associated with reduced levels of physical functioning, limitations in physical role activities, and decreased social functioning. Respiratory symptom burden contributed to models of physical functioning, general health perceptions, and vitality and fatigue. These results are similar to the finding of Ruffin and colleagues [7] of the importance of symptom burden in predicting QOL of patients with chronic lung disease. Phlegm and the combination of cough and phlegm were related to bodily pain and general health, respectively. The objective assessment of pulmonary function did not significantly contribute to any of the dimensions of QOL. These findings underscore the importance of subjective perceptions of symptoms, in addition to objective measures of pulmonary function, as has been reported by studies of patients with chronic lung diseases [7–10]. In particular, dyspnea in relationship to physical function is commonly reported in the setting of advanced lung cancer [38]. As reported in other studies [7–9], QOL ratings did not always correlate with the severity of pulmonary functional impairment or even the severity of symptoms [39].

Quality of life in lung cancer compared with other cancers

In 1994, Schag and colleagues [40] reported that lung cancer survivors experience more physical and psychosocial problems than survivors of colon or prostate cancer. In their analysis, the length of survival was not associated with QOL ratings in lung cancer patients; however, only five long-term lung cancer (LTLC) survivors were included in the study [40]. Some analyses of large population-based cancer survivor cohorts [41–43] have suggested that lung cancer survivors experience a heavy burden of illness that may persist for a prolonged period of time. QOL was evaluated in a patient cohort that was identified from the 1998 National Health Information Survey [41] including 54 lung cancer survivors, 92 melanoma survivors, 377 breast cancer survivors, and 169 colon cancer survivors. Health utility as measured by the Health and Activities Limitation Index was assessed according to the time from diagnosis in acute periods (ie, 1 year); short-term periods (ie, 1–5 years); and long-term periods (ie, 5 years). The mean health utility score in lung cancer survivors was lowest (indicating the worst QOL) among all cancer sites, and for both acute and long-term periods [41]. In this study, 20 individuals were LTLC survivors. Hewitt and colleagues [42] reported the health and disability status among 4878 cancer survivors. Relative to female breast cancer survivors, survivors of lung and respiratory (larynx and pharynx) cancer reported significantly poorer general health status and were bothered by more psychologic problems [42]. Yabroff and colleagues [43] compared the general health status, limitations in activity, and health utility among 1823 cancer survivors and 5469 matched control subjects who were also identified from the National Health Information Survey. Cancer survivors had poorer health outcomes when compared with control subjects, and the measures of illness burden in cancer survivors remained similar regardless of the interval since diagnosis. Lung cancer survivors, when combined with survivors of esophagus, liver, pancreas, and stomach cancer, reported greater illness burden than the survivors of cancers in all other sites [43].

Quality of life in long-term lung cancer survivors

The evaluation of QOL with particular focus on LTLC survivors has been limited to that of a few cross-sectional cohorts [36,41,44,45]. Sarna and colleagues [36,44–46] evaluated the demographic and clinical characteristics and QOL among 142 NSCLC patients who had survived for a minimum of 5 years. The investigators used the Quality of Life-Cancer Survivors tool and the SF-36 to measure QOL outcomes, and the Center for Epidemiologic Studies depression scale to assess distressed mood as a risk factor for poor QOL. Although most survivors self-reported that they were in "good" general health, QOL varied widely. When compared with published aggregate norm scores of the SF-36 physical component and mental component for a sample of older adults [44], lung cancer survivors scored similarly in both measures. Seventy percent of survivors reported their general health status as "good to excellent," despite 70% having comorbid medical conditions, 52% having impaired pulmonary function, and 66% having existing respiratory symptoms [41,42]. Greater than 70% of the participants described themselves as hopeful, and 50% of participants viewed their cancer experience as contributing to their positive life changes (as determined by the Quality of Life-Cancer Survivors tool) [44].

Twenty-one percent of the survivors, however, were restricted largely to bed rest and 11% could not leave the house because of severe respiratory symptoms [36]. Approximately 25% of patients felt fatigue or were bothered by aches or pain. Twenty-two percent scored more than 16 on the Center for Epidemiologic Studies depression scale, 28 indicating significant depressive symptoms or distressed mood. In a multivariable assessment, distressed mood was found to be a significant and major predictor of a worse score for all three QOL measures (ie, Quality of Life-Cancer Survivors tool global score, and SF-36 physical component and mental component).

For the SF-36 physical component, older age and having more comorbid conditions were significantly associated with a diminished QOL [44]. In a separate multivariable assessment of QOL including respiratory symptoms, the presence of dyspnea had a significant impact on QOL subscales as measured by the SF-36 physical component and mental component. It was reported that comorbid unstable angina was positively associated with severe distress caused by dyspnea. Other factors significantly influencing QOL were the total number of comorbidities, the total number of respiratory symptoms, and marital status [36].

Evangelista and colleagues [45] evaluated health risk behaviors including smoking, exposure to second-hand smoke, alcohol consumption, and weight control (overweight) in the same cohort. Eighteen percent of patients were currently smoking, 58% consumed alcohol, and 51% were overweight at the time of the survey. All risk behaviors were associated with a perceived poor health status, and the authors addressed the need to promote lifestyle changes to improve QOL. A subsample of participants from the parent cohort [36,44,45] were interviewed, and such issues as change in conception of life, awareness of health and self-care, changes in physical ability, adjustment to changes, and appreciation and willingness to give back for received support were recognized as important to their QOL. Survivors expressed themselves differentially (ie, positive versus negative) on these issues when grouped into those with distressed mood and those without distressed mood. Demographic and clinical factors, such as age, gender, cancer histology, treatment, and time since diagnosis, between the two groups were similar; mean scores for the SF-36 physical component and mental component were both lower, and comorbidity was more common among those in the distressed-mood group [46].

Twenty LTLC survivors were included in a separate cross-sectional evaluation of QOL within a larger cancer survivor cohort [41]. When the mean health utility score among LTLC survivors was compared with that of lung cancer survivors within the first year of diagnosis, LTLC survivors scored substantially higher (by 47%); however, this was not a longitudinal evaluation of the same patients over time, and the results may be biased. In a multiple regression model evaluating predictors of health utility in LTLC survivors, the presence of pain or a history of angina had significant negative impact on the measured outcomes [41].

Clinical events that may influence long-term health and quality of life among lung cancer survivors

Lung cancer treatment

The long-term adverse consequence of cancer treatment has received limited attention among patients with adult-onset cancers [47]. Especially in lung cancer patients, the high mortality rate has made it difficult adequately to assess treatment-related late toxicity [48]. The association between treatment modalities and QOL has not been assessed in LTLC survivors, and no studies have evaluated longitudinal changes of QOL in patients following treatment for their lung cancer over a period of 2 years [17,19,23,32,49,50].

Quality of life and lung cancer surgery

Patients with lung cancer frequently have some degree of lung function impairment [51]. Although lung resection remains the most effective treatment for patients with operable NSCLC [52,53], patients with borderline lung function are at increased risk of functional impairment postoperatively. For many patients, the risk of an impaired HRQOL after surgery is an important consideration when deciding whether to proceed with surgery. Some patients may regard immediate postoperative complications as an acceptable risk, but are not prepared to accept significant postoperative functional debility [54]. Some, however, suggested otherwise; if patients received curable resection and have got cured, it seems that they would almost all be satisfied with their postoperative QOL [55]. There is very little information available about the effect of surgery on HRQOL in this group of patients, and the way in which postoperative HRQOL relates to preoperative factors [55].

The long-term goals of lung cancer surgery include improved length and QOL [49]. The main focus for clinicians is predicted mortality and morbidity, but patients are concerned about potential long-term disability [54]. Follow-up of patients with lung cancer to include both survival and postoperative QOL may offer a more comprehensive approach to evaluating the associated risks and benefits [55,56].

There are few published reports of HRQOL in surgical patients [17,57]. Using the generic SF-36 questionnaire, preoperative functional health status in lung cancer surgical patients was significantly impaired, and that pain and impaired functioning persisted for 6 months [58]. Another study of 117 patients undergoing thoracotomy showed that patients with cancer reported dyspnea four times as often as patients with benign disease, and that QOL returned to preoperative levels by 6 to 9 months [17]. Zieren and colleagues [19] found that although HRQOL deteriorated soon after surgery, it was restored within 3 to 6 months in disease-free patients. HRQOL in long-term survivors of NSCLC showed a hopeful attitude and patients viewed lung cancer as having made a positive change in their lives [44]. Another study of selected surgical lung cancer patients showed significant benefit in terms of long-term QOL [59].

One study [23] showed that potentially operable patients had acceptable preoperative HRQOL. Compared with the general population, however, a candidate for lung resection with lung cancer had worse QOL [60]. Most patients did not experience pain, anorexia, constipation, diarrhea, nausea, or vomiting, although fatigue, dyspnea, and cough were reported with most suffering a mild to moderate degree. In common with other studies, most of the patients had recovered by 3 months follow-up [19,60]. Dales and colleagues [17] studied prospectively the QOL in lung cancer patients following surgical resection through thoracotomy; they found that QOL deteriorated in the first 3 months after surgery but returned to preoperative levels at 6 to 9 months. Similar findings were reported by Zieren and colleagues [19] in a more recent study.

Win and colleagues [23] indicated that cough was reduced immediately after operation most probably because of postoperative pain interfering with the cough reflex. Hemoptysis had resolved in all patients after surgery. Although only a minority of patients suffered from this, it was the most frightening for them and its resolution was a positive change in their life. Financial difficulty was reported in only 6%, mostly those who were self-employed and unable to work around the time of operation.

Several studies have shown that physical domains of QOL deteriorate early after lung cancer surgery but improve to baseline by 6 months after surgery [17,19,23]. To the contrary, Mangione and colleagues [50] reported a persistently declining perception of general health, vitality, physical function, and bodily pain at 12 months after surgery. The survivors' perception of symptoms was important to QOL, implying the need for monitoring respiratory symptoms after a thoracotomy [36]. Chronic pain is the most common complication after lung cancer surgery and, indeed, was one of the most commonly reported problems among LTLC survivors [44]. A usually mild but chronic pain after lung cancer surgery is known as the "postthoracotomy pain syndrome" and is seen in up to 80% of patients following a thoracotomy, with severe and disabling pain occurring in 5% [61]. Pain can last for more than 4 years in approximately 30% of patients [62].

Some concentrate on QOL and prediction of surgical outcome. Whether preoperative comorbidity and physiologic data could predict QOL after surgery was also an important issue. Win and colleagues [23] found no significant association between preoperative HRQOL scales and poor outcome as defined by surgical mortality or major complication. This is compatible with previous studies [17]. One previous study, however, found that QOL was the strongest prognostic factor for survival in lung cancer patients [63]. QOL measures had poor correlation with forced expiratory volume in 1 second, transfer coefficient (KCO), and exercise capacity in one recent study [60]. The study by Win and colleagues [23] did, however, show a weak correlation between the preoperative percentage predicted transfer capacity of lung for carbon monoxide (TLCO) and postoperative HRQOL, which supports the findings of a previous study [58]. This could possibly be caused by chance as a result of the multiple analyses performed, or if it is a real association, could be explained by the fact that TLCO may be the most representative measure of the extent of underlying lung disease, being affected by the severity of underlying emphysema, associated underlying interstitial fibrosis, or pulmonary hypertension. Functional variables cannot substitute for specific evaluation of QOL. Brunelli and colleagues [60] found the most interesting and encouraging finding that patients traditionally considered at higher risk for surgery had postoperative physical and emotional QOL similar to those observed in younger and fitter patients.

Preoperative global health status, physical function, and cognitive function were significantly correlated with 6-month postoperative global health status [23]. Dyspnea and dysphagia on the lung cancer module questionnaire and fatigue, pain, and diarrhea on the QLQ-C30 questionnaire were significantly inversely correlated with 6-month postoperative global health status, most probably because these symptoms closely represent late stage of disease.

Quality of life in different types of lung cancer surgery

Nomori and colleagues [64] recently reported no significant differences between their video-assisted thoracic surgery group and an anterior thoracotomy group for lung cancer resection in terms of postoperative respiratory muscle strength, 6-minute walk test, and pain scores after 2 weeks. It should be noted, however, that in their video-assisted thoracic surgery group rib spreading was used [65]. Landreneau and colleagues [66] studied the prevalence of chronic pain and pain-related morbidity after pulmonary resection comparing video-assisted thoracic surgery with thoracotomy; they found that video-assisted thoracic surgery is associated with reduced pain and shoulder dysfunction during the first year after surgery. No significant differences could be found, however, after a year follow-up. Possible QOL benefits of video-assisted thoracic surgery are likely to be maximal up to 9 months postoperatively. Sugiura and colleagues [67] assessed the long-term QOL in lung cancer patients following surgery, however, comparing video-assisted thoracic surgery with thoracotomy; they found that video-assisted thoracic surgery was associated with long-term QOL benefits. Overall, this study [68] shows that the predictors that positively affected the physical components of QOL were better performance in forced vital capacity and 6-minute walk test and less extensive lung resections.

The degree of lung resection (pneumonectomy, lobectomy, sleeve resection, segmental wedge resection) has been associated with varying degrees of pulmonary and functional status compromise [17–19]. Pulmonary function assessment alone, however, has been a poor predictor of patients' perceptions of physical disruptions in day-to-day activities [20,21].

Quality of life and radiotherapy

The occurrence of clinical pneumonitis and changes in pulmonary function are well-known adverse effects of radiation therapy. Radiation pneumonitis, defined as grade 2 or higher according to the South-West Oncology Group toxicity criteria [69,70], was reported in 15% to 20% of lung cancer patients receiving external-beam radiotherapy. The results suggested older age, low performance status, low pulmonary function, high radiotherapy dose, and chemotherapy exposure as possible risk factors [69–71].

To evaluate the relative influence of the late toxicity of radiotherapy on long-term survival, Machtay and colleagues [72] calculated the risk of death from intercurrent disease following postoperative radiotherapy in NSCLC patients. Age and radiotherapy dose were marginally associated with a higher risk of death from intercurrent disease; however, the actuarial survival rate at 4 years was only minimally decreased when compared with a matched population [73].

Quality of life and chemotherapy

Many chemotherapy agents cause cardiopulmonary or other toxicities, and several studies [73,74] have suggested a higher risk of perioperative complications when chemotherapy is administered before pulmonary resection. Information is scarce regarding the long-term adverse effects of chemotherapy in lung cancer patients.

Comorbidity

In general, cancer survivors with other comorbid conditions (comorbidity) possess a 5- to 10-times higher likelihood of poor health and disability when compared with individuals without a history of cancer or other chronic diseases [42]. In older cancer survivors, the presence of comorbidity was significantly correlated with impaired functional status regardless of the period of time from their cancer diagnosis [75]. The prevalence and severity of comorbidity has been reported to be especially high in lung cancer patients compared with survivors of other cancer sites [76,77]. The relative impact of comorbidity on 1-year survival was among the lowest, however, and was disproportionate to the survival rates [78].

Although most studies report a detrimental effect, the reported relative impact of comorbidity on lung cancer survival is not consistent among studies [79–81] and may be influenced by the different methods of data collection or by the use of different assessment tools [81]. Although the relative impact of comorbidity on survival in LTLC survivors is largely unknown, the frequency of comorbid conditions was significantly related to both the physical and mental health domains of QOL [44]. Comorbid angina was a cause of adverse influence on QOL among LTLC survivors in two studies [36,41].

The impact of multiple factors that influence medical complications and QOL in LTLC survivors needs to be better characterized individually and in combination. The significance of the interaction between aging-related comorbidities and frailty, and the adverse effects of lung cancer therapy, smoking, and their relationship with the vulnerability for subsequent death or other causes of health deterioration are largely unknown [47]. An understanding of these factors will allow precise risk estimation for efficient disease prevention strategies. One of the most important, and also challenging, steps is to establish a representative patient population to allow multidimensional research [47], which enables the assessment of a longitudinal change in QOL and allows for an estimation of significant predictors of QOL in their relationship to different time points in survivorship. Finally, intervention research on behavioral changes should be promoted to generate accurate knowledge and to develop long-term management and intervention strategies.

Late recurrence and new primary cancers

Cancer recurrence and the occurrence of new primary cancers are life-threatening clinical events that plague the course of lung cancer survivors. Although noting the difficulty in differential diagnosis, many studies [82,83] have evaluated the occurrence of these events.

Although late recurrence has been reported more than 10 years after an initial diagnosis of NSCLC [84], most recurrences are detected within 2 years after the patient undergoes surgical resection [85]. Several studies [84–87] have reported a 4% to 5% prevalence of recurrent disease in 5-year survivors following surgical resection. Two cohorts [85,88] of disease-free 5-year survivors of stage I NSCLC have reported an incidence rate of 2% to 3% per patient-year. Lung cancer survivors are at an increased risk of the development of subsequent primary cancers, including those of the lung. Johnson and colleagues [89] summarized that the risk of developing second lung cancers and other aerodigestive tumors in treated lung cancer patients is approximately 10-fold higher than that of adult smokers. The occurrence of subsequent primary lung cancer in patients undergoing surgical resection for NSCLC has been estimated to be 1% to 2% per patient-year [89]. The incidence of subsequent primary lung cancer was reported to increase twofold after 5 years of surgery when compared with 5 years after surgery [85]. The cumulative risk of subsequent primary lung cancer or other smoking-related cancers reaches 13% to 20% at 6 to 8 years after the patient undergoes resection of NSCLC [89]. An especially high risk of the development of subsequent primary lung cancer has been reported in patients with treated SCLC [89]. The risk per patient-year has been reported to increase from 2% to 13% after the passage of more than 10 years. The cumulative risk of the development of subsequent primary lung cancer results in a striking 30% at 10 to 12 years after the initial treatment [87]. Chest radiotherapy and continued smoking were found significantly to increase this risk [90].

Overall and disease-specific survival

Limited information is available regarding long-term survival rates among lung cancer patients at the population level. Wingo and colleagues [91] reported survival rates at 5, 10, and 15 years among patients with breast, prostate, colon and rectum, and lung malignancies who received diagnoses from 1974 to 1991, based on data collected by the SEER program. The relative survival rates were calculated by dividing the observed survival rates for each cancer diagnosis by the survival rates of the general United States population with the same gender, race, and age characteristics. Unique to lung cancer survivors was an apparent trend in relative survival in which a higher age at diagnosis was positively associated with a worse survival rate, regardless of race, gender, stage, or length of follow-up. When conditional relative survival rates (ie, the 5-year survival rate among LTLC survivors relative to matched subjects) were calculated in 5- and 10-year survivors of lung cancer, they were approximately 10% to 30% lower than the same measures observed in other cancer survivors [91]. The results indicate that even after LTLC long-term survival, lung cancer patients are still substantially vulnerable to the risks of death from all causes and that elderly survivors have a more pronounced risk.

Favorable disease-specific survival in NSCLC patients has been described in two large cohorts of 5-year survivors following surgical resection [87,92]. Martini and colleagues [87] followed 686 5-year disease-free survivors of NSCLC in resected stage I-IIIA. The estimated 10-year survival rate, when accounting only for lung cancer–related deaths, was 92.4%. Okada and colleagues [92] reported a similar 10-year survival rate of 91% in 421 5-year survivors. Martini and colleagues [87] reported that among the 369 5-year survivors, 76 had died before 10 years; 18 (24% of all causes of death) from lung malignancy and 58 (76%) from other causes. Other studies [84,93,94] have reported lung malignancy to account for 29% to 49% of all deaths noted among 5-year survivors of NSCLC following surgical resection; however, follow-up time varied among these studies.

The survival characteristics beyond 5 years in patients receiving nonsurgical treatment for NSCLC have been documented in limited reports. In a follow-up study [95] of 49 5-year survivors after undergoing radical radiation therapy for NSCLC, the overall actuarial 10-year survival rate was 65%. Among patients who were free from disease progression at 5 years, 81% remained free from disease progression at between 5 and 10 years [95]. Long-term follow-up data from clinical trials that evaluated the role of combined chemotherapy-radiation in the treatment of unresectable NSCLC were reported by two groups [96,97]. The estimated survival rates for the study arm receiving combined-modality treatment were 19% at 5 years and 13% at 7 years in the Cancer and Leukemia Group B 8433 trial [96], and were 14% at 5 years and 12% at 7 years in the six Japan Clinical Oncology Group trials [97]. In the latter study [97], the authors noted no deaths after 7 years following treatment.

Lung cancer survivors do not experience the same length of life and QOL as their age-matched peers or other cancer survivors. Lung cancer patients fare less well than survivors of other cancers because of the nature of the cancer and the predominant smoking history of most of the patients. There is clearly a need to identify and intervene with subgroups of patients who are at an elevated risk of premature death and diminished QOL.

Because the aging of the population is inevitable, survivors of lung cancer, especially those who are elderly, should receive continuous attention regarding their health and QOL beyond the expected cure of their primary cancer. Advanced age is associated with other chronic health problems; the assessment of comorbid conditions is extremely important and should be carefully conducted [98,99]. Methodologies in comorbidity assessment among lung cancer survivors call for further development [52,83]. Little information is available on the assessment of the late effects of cancer treatment in lung cancer survivors. A change in standard patient management, including the wider application of multimodality treatment options, may or may not influence the significance of the issue of the possible late side effects of treatment. The occurrence of secondary cancers is an important health matter among LTLC survivors. These events should be further evaluated for risk factors, including the genetic and molecular effects of smoking and lung cancer treatment and the susceptibility possessed by the host and primary tumor.

Summary

Several studies have shown that physical domains of QOL deteriorate early after lung cancer surgery but improve to baseline by 6 months after surgery. Impaired cardiopulmonary function following pulmonary resection is an important predictor of immediate postoperative morbidity; meanwhile, an objective assessment of pulmonary function did not significantly contribute to QOL in LTLC survivors. Chronic pain is the most common complication after lung cancer surgery. Lung cancer survivors do not experience the same length of life and QOL as their age-matched peers or other cancer survivors. Lung cancer patients are less well than survivors of other cancers because of the nature of the cancer and the smoking history. There is clearly a need to identify and intervene with subgroups of patients who are at an elevated risk of premature death and diminished QOL.

References

[1] Karnofsky DA, Burchenal JH. Evaluation of chemotherapeutic agents. In: Macload CM, editor. The clinical evaluation of chemotherapeutic agents in cancer. New York: Columbia U. Press; 1949. p. 191–205.

[2] Priestman TJ, Baum M. Evaluation of quality of life in patients receiving treatment for advanced breast cancer. Lancet 1976;1:899–910.

[3] Schag AS, Heinrich RL. Development of a comprehensive quality of life measurement tool: CARES. Oncology 1990;4:135–8.

[4] Ishitani K. Cancer and quality of life: concept of QOL. Tokyo: Life Science; 1991. p. 4–18.

[5] Schipper H, Clinch J, McMurray A, et al. Measuring the quality of life of cancer patients. The functional living index-cancer: development and validation. J Clin Oncol 1984;2:472–83.

[6] Ries LAG, Kosary CL, Hankey BF, et al. Lung and bronchus cancer: SEER cancer statistics review, 1973–1996. Bethesda (MD): National Cancer Institute; 1999.

[7] Ruffin RE, Wilson DH, Chittleborough AM, et al. Multiple respiratory symptoms predict quality of life in chronic lung disease: a population-based study of Australian adults. Qual Life Res 2000;9:1031–9.

[8] Mahler DA, Faryniarz K, Tomlinson D, et al. Impact of dyspnea and physiologic function on general health status in patients with chronic obstructive pulmonary disease. Chest 1992;102:395–401.

[9] Mahler DA, Jones PW. Measurement of dyspnea and quality of life in advanced lung disease. Clin Chest Med 1997;18:457–69.

[10] Chang JA, Curtis JR, Patrick DL, et al. Assessment of health-related quality of life in patients with interstitial lung disease. Chest 1999;116:1175–82.

[11] Dudgeon DJ, Rosenthal S. Management of dyspnea and cough in patients with cancer: pain and palliative care. Hematol Oncol Clin North Am 1996;10: 157–70.

[12] Gore JM, Brophy CJ, Greenstone MA. How well do we care for patients with end stage chronic obstructive pulmonary disease. Thorax 2000;55:1000–6.

[13] Dockery DW, Speizer FE, Ferris BG, et al. Cumulative and reversible effects of lifetime smoking on simple tests of lung function in adults. Am Rev Respir Dis 1988;137:286–92.

[14] Pelkonen M, Notkola IL, Tukiainen H, et al. Smoking cessation, decline in pulmonary function and total mortality: a 30 year follow up study among the Finnish cohorts of the Seven Countries Study. Thorax 2001;56:703–7.

[15] Gritz ER. Smoking and smoking cessation in cancer patients. Br J Addict 1991;86:549–54.

[16] Ferguson MK, Skosey C, Hoffman PC, et al. Sex associated differences in presentation and survival in patients with lung cancer. J Clin Oncol 1990;8:1402–7.

[17] Dales R, Belanger R, Shamji F, et al. Quality of life following thoracotomy for lung cancer. J Clin Epidemiol 1994;47:1443–9.

[18] Nugent AM, Steele IC, Carragher AM, et al. Effect of thoracotomy and lung resection on exercise capacity in patients with lung cancer. Thorax 1999;54:34–8.

[19] Zieren HU, Muller JM, Hamberger U, et al. Quality of life after surgical therapy of bronchogenic carcinoma. Eur J Cardiothorac Surg 1996;10:233–7.

[20] Larsen KR, Svendsen UG, Milman N, et al. Cardiopulmonary function at rest and during exercise after resection for bronchial carcinoma. Ann Thorac Surg 1997;64:960–4.

[21] Bolliger CT, Jordan P, Soler M, et al. Pulmonary function and exercise capacity after lung resection. Eur Respir J 1996;9:415–21.

[22] Montazeri A, Gillis CR, McEwen J. Quality of life in patients with lung cancer: a review of literature from 1970–1995. Chest 1998;113:467–81.

[23] Win T, Sharples L, Wells FC, et al. Effect of lung cancer surgery on quality of life. Thorax 2005;60:234–8.

[24] Balduyck B, Hendriks J, Lauwers P, et al. Quality of life evolution after lung cancer surgery: a prospective study in 100 patients. Lung Cancer 2007;56(3):423–31 [Epub: 2007 Feb 16].

[25] Nonaka M, Ohno M, Fukuzumi M, et al. [Quality of life of long-term survivors of surgically treated lung cancer]. Kyobu Geka 2006;59(7):519–28 [in Japanese].

[26] Brown J, Thorpe H, Napp V, et al. Assessment of quality of life in the supportive care setting of the big lung trial in non-small-cell lung cancer. J Clin Oncol 2005;23(30):7417–27.

[27] Lübbe AS, Krischke NR, Dimeo F, et al. Health-related quality of life and pulmonary function in lung cancer patients undergoing medical rehabilitation treatment. Wien Med Wochenschr 2001;151(1–2):29–34.

[28] Bruley DK. Beyond reliability and validity: analysis of selected quality-of-life instruments for use in palliative care. J Palliat Med 1999;2(3):299–309.

[29] Nicklasson M, Bergman B. Validity, reliability and clinical relevance of EORTC QLQ-C30 and LC13 in patients with chest malignancies in a palliative setting. Qual Life Res 2007;16(6):1019–28.

[30] Long H, Lin ZC, Lin YB, et al. [Quality of life after lobectomy for early stage non-small cell lung cancer: video-assisted thoracoscopic surgery versus minimal incision thoracotomy]. Ai Zheng 2007;26(6):624–8 [in Chinese].

[31] Hollen PJ, Gralla RJ, Rittenberg CN. Quality of life as a clinical trial endpoint: determining the appropriate interval for repeated assessments in patients with advanced lung cancer. Support Care Cancer 2004;12(11):767–73.

[32] Myrdal G, Valtysdottir S, Lambe M, et al. Quality of life following lung cancer surgery. Thorax 2003;58(3):194–7.

[33] Barlesi F, Doddoli C, Loundou A, et al. Preoperative psychological global well being index (PGWBI) predicts postoperative quality of life for patients with non-small cell lung cancer managed with thoracic surgery. Eur J Cardiothorac Surg 2006;30(3):548–53.

[34] Paull DE, Thomas ML, Meade GE, et al. Determinants of quality of life in patients following pulmonary resection for lung cancer. Am J Surg 2006;192(5):565–71.

[35] Cooley M. Patterns of symptom distress in adults receiving treatment for lung cancer. J Palliat Care 2002;18:150–9.

[36] Sarna L, Evangelista L, Tashkin D, et al. Impact of respiratory symptoms and pulmonary function on quality of life of long-term survivors of non-small cell lung cancer. Chest 2004;125:439–45.

[37] Bergman B, Aaronson NK. Quality-of-life and cost-effectiveness assessment in lung cancer. Curr Opin Oncol 1995;7:138–43.

[38] Tanaka K, Akechi T, Okuyama T, et al. Impact of dyspnea, pain, and fatigue on daily life activities in ambulatory patients with advanced lung cancer. J Pain Symptom Manage 2002;23:417–23.

[39] Dales RE, Spitzer WO, Schecter MT, et al. The influence of psychological status on respiratory symptom reporting. Am Rev Respir Dis 1989;139:1459–63.

[40] Schag CAC, Ganz PA, Wing DS, et al. Quality of life in adult survivors of lung, colon, and prostate cancer. Qual Life Res 1994;3:127–41.

[41] Ko CY, Maggard M, Livingstone EH. Evaluating health utility in patients with melanoma, breast cancer, colon cancer, and lung cancer: a nation-wide population-based assessment. J Surg Res 2003;114: –5.

[42] Hewitt M, Rowland JH, Yancik R. Cancer survivors in the United States: age, health, and disability. J Gerontol A Biol Sci Med Sci 2003;58:82–91.

[43] Yabroff KR, Lawrence WF, Clauser S, et al. Burden of illness in cancer survivors: findings from a population-based national survey. J Natl Cancer Inst 2004;96:1322–30.

[44] Sarna L, Padilla G, Holmes C, et al. Quality of life of long-term survivors of non-small-cell lung cancer. J Clin Oncol 2002;20:2920–9.

[45] Evangelista LS, Sarna L, Brecht ML, et al. Health perceptions and risk behaviors of lung cancer survivors. Heart Lung 2003;32:131–9.
[46] Maliski SL, Sarna L, Evangelista L, et al. The aftermath of lung cancer-balancing the good and bad. Cancer Nurs 2003;26:237–43.
[47] Ganz PA. Why and how to study the fate of cancer survivors: observations from the clinic and the research laboratory. Eur J Cancer 2003;39:2136–41.
[48] Bonner JA, Tincher SA, Fiveash JB. Balancing the possible effectiveness of postoperative radiotherapy for non-small cell lung cancer against the possible detriment of radiation induced toxicity. J Clin Oncol 2001;19:3905–7.
[49] Handy JR, Asaph JW, Skokan L, et al. What happens to patients undergoing lung cancer surgery? Outcomes and quality of life before and after surgery. Chest 2002;122:21–30.
[50] Mangione CM, Goldman L, Orav EJ, et al. Health-related quality of life after elective surgery: measurement of longitudinal changes. J Gen Intern Med 1997;12:686–97.
[51] Legge JS, Palmer KN. Pulmonary function in bronchial carcinoma. Thorax 1973;28:588–91.
[52] Reif MS, Socinski MA, Rivera MP. Evidence-based medicine in the treatment of non-small-cell lung cancer. Clin Chest Med 2000;21:107–20.
[53] Pearson FG. Current status of surgical resection for lung cancer. Chest 1994;106:337S–9S.
[54] Cykert S, Kissling G, Hansen CJ. Patient preferences regarding possible outcomes of lung resection: what outcomes should preoperative evaluations target? Chest 2000;117:1551–9.
[55] Aaronson NK, Ahmedzai S, Bullinger M. The EORTC core quality of life questionnaire: interim results of an international field study. In: Osoba D, editor. The effect of cancer on quality of life. Boca Raton: CRC Press; 1991.
[56] Denton TA, Matloff JM. Optimizing cardiothoracic surgery information for a managed care environment. Ann Thorac Surg 1995;60:1522–5.
[57] Dales RE, Dionne G, Leech JA, et al. Preoperative prediction of pulmonary complications following thoracic surgery. Chest 1993;104:155–9.
[58] Aaronson NK, Ahmedzai S, Bergman B, et al. The European organization for research and treatment of cancer QLQ-C30: a quality-of-life instrument for use in international clinical trials in oncology. J Natl Cancer Inst 1993;85:365–76.
[59] Pompeo E, De Dominicis E, Ambrogi V, et al. Quality of life after tailored combined surgery for stage I non-small-cell lung cancer and severe emphysema. Ann Thorac Surg 2003;76:1821–7.
[60] Brunelli A, Socci L, Refai M, et al. Quality of life before and after major lung resection for lung cancer: a prospective follow-up analysis. Ann Thorac Surg 2007;84(2):410–6.
[61] Ruckdeschel JC, Piantadosi S. Quality of life in lung cancer surgical adjuvant trials. Chest 1994;106: 324S–8S.
[62] Rogers ML, Duffy JP. Surgical aspects of chronic postthoracotomy pain. Eur J Cardiothorac Surg 2000;18:711–6.
[63] Karmakar MK, Ho AM. Postthoracotomy pain syndrome. Thorac Surg Clin 2004;14:345–52.
[64] Nomori H, Horio H, Naruke T, et al. What is the advantage of a thoracoscopic lobectomy over a limited thoracotomy procedure for lung cancer surgery? Ann Thorac Surg 2001;72:879–84.
[65] Yim AP, Landreneau RJ, Izzat MB, et al. Is video-assisted thoracoscopic lobectomy a unified approach? Ann Thorac Surg 1998;66:1155–8.
[66] Landreneau RJ, Mack MJ, Hazelrigg SR, et al. Prevalence of chronic pain after pulmonary resection by thoracotomy or video-assisted thoracic surgery. Thorac Cardiovasc Surg 1994;107:1079–86.
[67] Sugiura H, Morikawa T, Kaji M, et al. Long-term benefits for the quality of life after video-assisted thoracoscopic lobectomy in patients with lung cancer. Surg Laparosc Endosc Percutan Tech 1999;9:403–8.
[68] Li WWL, Lee TW, Lam SSY, et al. Quality of life following lung cancer resection: video assisted thoracic surgery vs thoracotomy. Chest 2002;122:584–9.
[69] Hernando ML, Marks LB, Bentel GC, et al. Radiation induced pulmonary toxicity: a dose-volume histogram analysis in 201 patients with lung cancer. Int J Radiat Oncol Biol Phys 2001;51:650–9.
[70] Rancati T, Ceresoli GL, Gagliardi G, et al. Factors predicting radiation pneumonitis in lung cancer patients: a retrospective study. Radiother Oncol 2003; 67:275–83.
[71] Robnett TJ, Machtay M, Vines EF, et al. Factors predicting severe radiation pneumonitis in patients receiving definitive chemoradiation for lung cancer. Int J Radiat Oncol Biol Phys 2000;48:89–94.
[72] Machtay M, Lee JH, Shrager JB, et al. Risk of death from intercurrent disease is not excessively increased by modern postoperative radiotherapy for high-risk resected non-small cell lung carcinoma. J Clin Oncol 2001;19:3912–7.
[73] Roberts JR, Eustis C, Devore R, et al. Induction chemotherapy increases perioperative complications in patients undergoing resection for non-small cell lung cancer. Ann Thorac Surg 2001;72:885–8.
[74] Leo F, Solli P, Spaggiari L, et al. Respiratory function changes after chemotherapy: an additional risk for postoperative respiratory complications? Ann Thorac Surg 2004;77:260–5.
[75] Garman KS, Pieper CF, Seo P, et al. Function in elderly cancer survivors depends on comorbidities. J Gerontol 2003;58A:1119–24.
[76] Piccirillo JF, Tierny RM, Costas I, et al. Prognostic importance of comorbidity in a hospital-based cancer registry. JAMA 2004;291:2441–7.

[77] Ogle KS, Swanson GM, Woods N, et al. Cancer and comorbidity: redefining chronic diseases. Cancer 2000;88:653–63.
[78] Read WL, Tierny RM, Page NC, et al. Differential prognostic impact of comorbidity. J Clin Oncol 2004;22:3099–103.
[79] Janssen-Heijen MLG, Smulders S, Lemmens VEPP, et al. Effect of comorbidity on the treatment and prognosis of elderly patients with non-small cell lung cancer. Thorax 2004;59:602–7.
[80] Battafarano RJ, Piccirillo JF, Meyers BF, et al. Impact of comorbidity on survival after surgical resection in patients with stage I non-small cell lung cancer. J Thorac Cardiovasc Surg 2002;123:280–7.
[81] Tammemagi CM, Neslund-Dudas C, Simoff M, et al. Impact of comorbidity on lung cancer survival. Int J Cancer 2003;103:792–802.
[82] Martini N, Melamed MR. Multiple primary lung cancers. J Thorac Cardiovasc Surg 1975;70:606–12.
[83] Rice D, Kim H-W, Sabichi A, et al. The risk of second primary tumors after resection of stage I non-small cell lung cancer. Ann Thorac Surg 2003;76:1001–8.
[84] Thomas PA, Rubinstein L. Malignant disease appearing late after operation for T1N0 non-small cell lung cancer. J Thorac Cardiovasc Surg 1993;106:1053–8.
[85] Martini N, Bains MS, Burt ME, et al. Incidence of local recurrence and second primary tumors in resected stage I lung cancer. J Thorac Cardiovasc Surg 1995;109:120–9.
[86] Immerman SC, Vanecko RM, Fry WA, et al. Site of recurrence in patients with stages I and II carcinoma of the lung resected for cure. Ann Thorac Surg 1981;32:23–7.
[87] Martini N, Rusch VW, Bains MS, et al. Factors influencing ten-year survival in resected stages I to IIIA non-small cell lung cancer. J Thorac Cardiovasc Surg 1999;117:32–8.
[88] Thomas P, Rubinstein L. Cancer recurrence after resection: T1N0 non-small cell lung cancer; Lung Cancer Study Group. Ann Thorac Surg 1990;49:242–6.
[89] Johnson BE, Cortazar P, Chute JP. Second lung cancers in patients successfully treated for lung cancer. Semin Oncol 1997;24:1–9.
[90] Tucker MA, Murray N, Shaw EG, et al. Second primary cancers related to smoking and treatment of small-cell lung cancer: lung cancer working cadre. J Natl Cancer Inst 1997;89:1782–8.
[91] Wingo PA, Ries LA, Parker SL, et al. Long-term cancer patient survival in the United States. Cancer Epidemiol Biomarkers Prev 1998;7:271–82.
[92] Okada M, Nishio W, Sakamoto T, et al. Long term survival and prognostic factors of five-year survivors with complete resection of non-small cell lung carcinoma. J Thorac Cardiovasc Surg 2003;126:558–62.
[93] Wada H, Fukuse T, Hitomi S. Long-term survival of surgical cases of lung cancer. Lung Cancer 1995;13:269–74.
[94] Rocco PM, Antkowiak JG, Takita H, et al. Long-term outcome after pneumonectomy for nonsmall cell lung cancer. J Surg Oncol 1996;61:278–80
[95] Mac Manus MP, Wada M, Matthews JP, et al. Characteristics of 49 patients who survived for 5 years following radical radiation therapy for non-small cell lung cancer: the potential for cure. Int J Radiat Oncol Biol Phys 2000;1:63–9.
[96] Dillman RO, Herndon J, Seagren SL, et al. Improved survival in stage III non-small cell lung cancer: seven-year follow-up of Cancer and Leukemia Group B (CALGB) 8433 trial. J Natl Cancer Inst 1996;88:1210–5.
[97] Ohe Y, Ishizuka N, Tamura T, et al. Long-term follow-up of patients with unresectable locally advanced non-small cell lung cancer treated with chemoradiotherapy: a retrospective analysis of the data from the Japan Clinical Oncology Group trials (JCOG0003A). Cancer Sci 2003;94:729–33.
[98] Yancik R, Ganz PA, Varricchio CG, et al. Perspectives on comorbidity and cancer in older patients: approaches to expand the knowledge base. J Clin Oncol 2001;19:1147–51.
[99] Ko C, Chaudhry S. The need for a multidisciplinary approach to cancer care. J Surg Res 2002;1C5:53–7.

ELSEVIER
SAUNDERS

Thorac Surg Clin 18 (2008) 93–105

THORACIC
SURGERY
CLINICS

Parenchymal-Sparing Resections: Why, When, and How

Matthew J. Schuchert, MD, Brian L. Pettiford, MD, James D. Luketich, MD, Rodney J. Landreneau, MD*

Division of Thoracic and Foregut Surgery, Heart, Lung and Esophageal Surgery Institute, University of Pittsburgh Medical Center, Shadyside Medical Building – Suite 715, P.O. Box 1, 5200 Centre Avenue, Pittsburgh, PA 15232, USA

The achievement of a complete surgical (R0) resection remains the hallmark principle guiding the therapy of patients who have early-stage (stage IA or IB) non-small cell lung cancer (NSCLC). Successful extirpation of the tumor with negative margins provides patients with the greatest chance of cure in the setting of stage I disease. To date, lobectomy remains the practice standard in patients who have acceptable cardiopulmonary function. The role of anatomic sublobar (segmental) resection as definitive management for early-stage NSCLC is evolving, however, and is gaining broader acceptance in patients who have small tumors (< 2 cm) and in those who have limited cardiopulmonary function or who might not tolerate conventional lobectomy. This article reviews the available data regarding the use of parenchymal-sparing resections in the setting of stage I NSCLC.

Historical perspective

The use of segmental resection was first reported by Churchill and Belsey [1] in 1939 for the management of bronchiectasis. The importance of individual control and division of the segmental bronchial and vascular structures during anatomic segmentectomy was well recognized [2] and was highlighted in Overholt and Langer's [3] treatise on the resection of each bronchopulmonary segment. Such early work established the use of anatomic segmentectomy as a valid option in the surgical treatment of discrete sublobar pathology.

At that time pneumonectomy was considered the only viable option in the surgical management of lung cancer [4]. Its attendant high morbidity and mortality (40%) led to the use of lobectomy as the preferred approach in the treatment of resectable NSCLC [5]. The use of anatomic segmentectomy for early-stage lung cancer was explored by some thoracic surgeons [6–9] and has been postulated to represent an adequate operation for early-stage lung cancer. The perceived complexity of this operative approach compared with lobectomy, however, and concerns regarding increased morbidity related to prolonged air leak and local recurrence rates have deterred most surgeons from using this approach for early-stage lung cancer [10]. The Lung Cancer Study Group (LCSG) conducted the only randomized study comparing sublobar resection with lobectomy for patients who had stage IA NSCLC [11]. The principal finding in this study was a threefold increase in local recurrence (17.2% versus 6.4%) in patients who had sublobar resection. Two years later, another prospective, multicenter, nonrandomized study demonstrated a similar trend for increased local recurrence in patients undergoing sublobar resection [12]. These are other

* Corresponding author.
E-mail address: landreneaurj@upmc.edu (R.J. Landreneau).

1547-4127/08/$ - see front matter
doi:10.1016/j.thorsurg.2007.11.007

studies have established lobectomy as the modern surgical approach of choice in patients who have early-stage lung cancer.

The increased identification of small NSCLC tumors by enhanced CT screening protocols in higher-risk surgical patients [13] has led many surgeons to question the appropriateness of lobectomy for these tumors (Fig. 1) [14,15]. A substantial body of literature from Japan and elsewhere has emerged during the last decade to produce a resurgence of interest in the use of anatomic segmentectomy for patients who have small peripheral NSCLC, especially those who otherwise might not tolerate lobectomy.

Box 1. Favorable criteria for anatomic segmentectomy

- Peripheral location (outer one third of the lung)
- Small tumors (< 2 cm in diameter)
- Pathologic margin greater than 1 cm (margin-to-tumor ratio > 1)
- Patient age over 75 years
- Marginal pulmonary function
- Ground-glass opacities; in situ carcinoma; bronchoalveolar cancer

Rationale for sublobar resection

The use of anatomic segmentectomy is generally accepted for the management of benign disease processes and metastatic carcinoma to the lung confined to an anatomic segment [1,16]. The use of sublobar resection (and segmentectomy in particular) has been accepted as a reasonable approach for resection of patients who have significant impairment in cardiopulmonary reserve [8]. The primary controversy over the years among thoracic surgeons has been with the use of segmentectomy as primary management of peripheral primary NSCLC in patients who are physiologically fit to undergo lobectomy.

Favorable criteria for the use of anatomic segmentectomy are listed in Box 1. Small (< 2 cm) tumors located peripherally within the lung parenchyma (the outer one third of the lung) represent lesions ideal for resection [17]. Such tumors permit the achievement of an adequate surgical margin (> 1 cm; margin-to-tumor size ratio > 1) with segmentectomy and are associated with a low rate of nodal involvement or distant metastases [18]. Anatomic segmentectomy certainly should be considered in elderly patients (> 75 years) and in those who have impaired pulmonary reserve [19,20]. In addition, this approach is recommended in patients who have small ground-glass opacities, which are associated with in situ carcinoma and early cancers with corresponding low local and distant recurrence rates [21].

Sublobar resections in such patients have been demonstrated to achieve lower perioperative morbidity and mortality rates [22,23] and to preserve pulmonary function compared with lobectomy

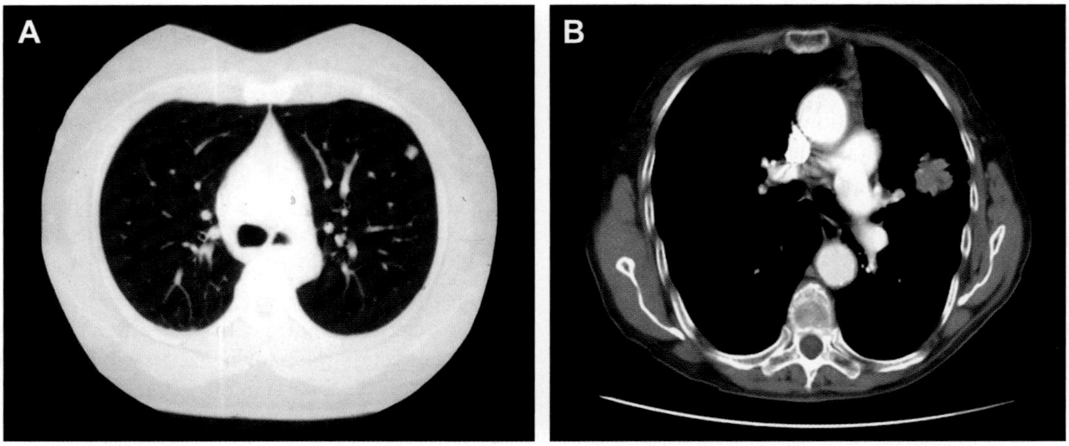

Fig. 1. CT images of (*A*) a small peripheral T1 lesion ideal for sublobar resection and (*B*) a larger, more centrally located lesion better treated with lobectomy.

[24,25]. Sublobular resection may be the only feasible surgical option in high-risk patients who have compromised cardiopulmonary function.

Preoperative evaluation

Most patients present to the thoracic surgeon with an abnormal nodule or mass lesion detected on chest CT scan. Isolated parenchymal lesions confined to segmental boundaries can be considered for segmental resection (Fig. 1A). Special attention should be focused on the mediastinum to rule out nodal involvement. Mediastinoscopy is performed, if indicated, based on enlarged mediastinal lymph nodes (> 1 cm in diameter) or fluorodeoxyglucose avidity on positron emission tomographic scanning [26,27]. CT scans should specifically include imaging of the liver and adrenal glands to exclude distant metastases. Brain MRI [28] and bone scanning [29] can be performed to exclude metastases in the presence of symptoms referable to these regions.

The thoracic surgeon also must evaluate carefully specific anatomic characteristics of the lesion being considered for sublobar resection. It generally is appreciated that lesions chosen for sublobar resection done either by open thoracotomy or video-assisted thorascopic surgery (VATS) approaches should be located within the outer third of the lung parenchyma, measure less than 3 cm in diameter, and have no evidence of endobronchial involvement during bronchoscopy (see Fig. 1). This approach minimizes the possibility of inadequate resection margins, staple-line dehiscence, and associated air leak or bleeding problems related to the distortion of the remaining lung parenchyma [18,30].

A complete physiologic evaluation of the patient being considered for sublobar resection is important. Usually the individual considered for sublobar resection is one whose cardiopulmonary functionality is in question. Thorough pulmonary functional evaluation is indicated. This evaluation must include formal pulmonary spirometry, arterial blood gas analysis, and assessment of carbon monoxide diffusion capacity. Based on spirometric data and general functional concerns, split-lung ventilation/perfusion nuclear scintigraphic assessment and maximum oxygen consumption exercise testing may be considered selectively before surgery. Cardiac functional assessment using standard or pharmacologic stress testing and two-dimensional echocardiography with estimates of pulmonary arterial pressures should be considered [31].

Surgical approaches and technical considerations

General principles

After intubation with a single-lumen endotracheal tube, a flexible bronchoscopy is performed in all patients to ensure the absence of endobronchial disease that would preclude the use of sublobar resection. A double-lumen tube then is inserted, and the thoracic surgeon confirms its position. These precautions can reduce the occurrence of time-consuming intraoperative problems associated with inadequate lung isolation. Sublobar resections generally are performed with the patient in the lateral decubitus position using either a VATS or thoracotomy approach.

Wedge versus segmentectomy

Sublobar resection for lung cancer can be performed with a simple wedge resection technique, with appropriate attention being paid to obtaining an adequate surgical margin. With the development of surgical stapling devices, this approach has become the dominant method of sublobar resection used today [19]. Most of the patients treated with sublobar resection in the LCSG study [11] as well as in the study by Landreneau and colleagues [12] underwent simple wedge resection. As discussed elsewhere, recurrence rates with sublobar wedge resections can be up to three times those seen with lobectomy with no apparent difference in 5-year survival [11,12,32].

In contrast, anatomic segmentectomy pays closer attention to a detailed anatomic bronchial and vascular dissection, with selective division of these structures in a manner analogous to the selective division of hilar structures performed in lobectomy. The addition of an extended parenchymal margin (extended segmentectomy) ensures the complete removal of the targeted anatomic segment with its vascular and lymphatic distribution. Theoretically, extended anatomic segmentectomy might permit a wider margin of resection than obtained with conventional wedge resection. For this approach to be successful, the tumor must conform to the resected segment and not be associated with nodal or distant metastases outside the resected distribution. In the LCSG trial segmental resection was shown to have a lower risk of local recurrence than a simple wedge resection [11] and may more closely approximate the results of lobectomy in terms of recurrence and survival. Okada and co-workers [33] published 5-year survival rates of 96.7% (tumors < 2 cm) and 84.6% (tumors 2–3 cm), which were superior to those of wedge resections (85.7% and 39.4%, respectively). In another study by El-Sherif and colleagues [34] evaluating 81 patients who had stage I NSCLC treated by either wedge resection (n = 55) or anatomic segmentectomy (n = 26), there was a significantly higher risk of locoregional recurrence with wedge resection (14/55, 25.5%) than with anatomic segmentectomy (1/26, 3.8%). Anatomic segmentectomy therefore may represent the ideal technique to minimize recurrence in situations where parenchyma-sparing techniques may be beneficial. When an adequate surgical margin is not obtainable with segmental resection, lobectomy should be performed.

Video-assisted thoracoscopic surgery versus open approach

Sublobar resection can be performed safely using either an open or VATS approach. The selection of the optimal approach in a given case depends on patient and tumor characteristics and on surgeon preference and experience. The VATS approach generally has been associated with reduced pain [35,36], shorter length of hospital stay [37,38], and fewer complications than open techniques [39], with equivalent oncologic outcomes [32,39]. The efficacy of the VATS approach with wedge resection has been well documented [14,18,35]. Formal thoracoscopic segmentectomy also has been performed with excellent results [40]. In the largest single-institution series published to date [39], 182 segmental resections were performed for stage I NSCLC (68 VATS; 114 open). There were no deaths in patients undergoing the VATS approach. VATS segmentectomy was associated with a shorter length of stay (5 versus 7 days) and lower infectious complication rate (3% versus 12%) than seen with the open surgery group. No difference was observed between the two groups in operative time, estimated blood loss, mortality, recurrence, or survival [39].

Whenever possible, the authors prefer to use the VATS approach to perform sublobar resection. When the appropriate lesion is selected for this approach, the VATS approach reduces hospital stay and postoperative infectious and pulmonary morbidity. An open approach is reserved for larger tumors or when exposure is difficult to achieve or maintain using a VATS approach.

Surgical technique: anatomic segmentectomy

In normal pulmonary anatomy, the right and left lungs are comprised of 19 bronchopulmonary segments, 10 on the right and 9 on the left. Each pulmonary segment consists of a sublobar bronchovascular unit and the corresponding pulmonary parenchyma that it supplies. Anatomic segmentectomy is the removal of one or more pulmonary parenchymal segments and the corresponding bronchovascular supply. In contradistinction, a nonanatomic or wedge resection is a sublobar resection without isolation and removal of the bronchovascular unit supplying the targeted lung parenchyma. When considering a segmental approach, it is critical to ensure that the residual lung parenchyma is of adequate size and conformation to merit the decision to perform a sublobar resection.

Open segmental resection is performed by either a muscle-sparing axillary thoracotomy or posterolateral mini-thoracotomy. The VATS approach is performed with a 10-mm camera port positioned in the seventh intercostal space along the mid-axillary line. A second posterior 10-mm port is placed along the same interspace in the posterior axillary line and is used for retraction and stapling. A 4-cm access incision is placed in the anterior axillary line at the level of the inframammary crease overlying the central portion of the hilum (Fig. 2). A 5-mm port is placed just inferior to the axillary hairline for additional instrumentation, as needed. Rib spreading is avoided. For each segment, selective isolation and division of the targeted bronchovascular pedicle is performed. To minimize the risk of bleeding and prolonged postoperative air leaks, the authors prefer the stapled, extended approach to segmentectomy, which incorporates the corresponding intersegmental veins, rather than a selective dissection and identification of the intersegmental

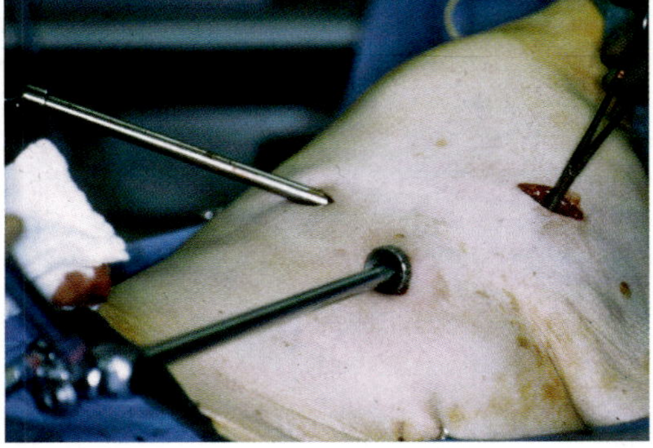

Fig. 2. Standard port incisions for VATS anatomic segmentectomy.

veins. Care is taken to inflate the lung partially before parenchymal resection to assist in identifying the appropriate boundaries of resection. Particular attention is paid to achieving an adequate surgical margin during the parenchymal division. The authors routinely sample N1 and N2 lymph nodes intraoperatively to evaluate for the possibility of occult nodal metastases.

Surgical technique: segmental pearls

Apical/apicoposterior segmentectomy. Division of the apical branch of the superior pulmonary vein is performed first and exposes the bifurcation of the superior division of the right pulmonary artery into the apical and anterior branches. The apical branch arises superiorly at this branch-point. Posterior to the artery courses the apical bronchus, which then is taken in succession. If the anatomic distinction of the bronchus is in doubt, clamping the specified bronchus with lung inflation can be useful before division.

Posterior segmentectomy. For posterior segmental resections, it frequently is useful to approach the bronchus first. The posterior bronchus is approached after incising the apical and posterior mediastinal pleura. The bronchus is taken first, followed by the posterior artery, which lies just anterior to the bronchus. When the major fissure is well developed, the posterior recurrent artery may be taken first, followed by the bronchus. The surgeon must be aware that a large proximal posterior artery can arise as a natural variant from the anterior-apical trunk and can course posterior to the bronchus. This variant can be identified when approaching the bronchus from the apicoposterior pleura and can be suspected when a diminutive posterior branch is encountered at the level of the fissure. In this case, the segmental pulmonary venous drainage to the posterior segment often is seen as several terminal branches of the interlobar pulmonary vein. Hemoclip ligation and division of these smaller branches can be performed readily before stapler ligation of the parenchyma at the segmental margin. Rarely, the posterior segmental artery may arise from the superior segmental artery, particularly if the latter vessel originates as a large trunk.

During left-sided posterior segmental resections, the primary concern following establishment of the interlobar plane and identification of the interlobar pulmonary artery is avoiding the division of high lingular arterial branches, which may be confused as accessory posterior segmental vasculature. After division of the posterior segmental artery or arteries, the posterior segmental bronchus can be palpated with blunt dissection. During the dissection of the left posterior segmental bronchus, it is important to avoid injury to the closely apposed venous drainage of the segment and the anterior and apical pulmonary segmental arteries anterior to it.

Anterior segmentectomy. The anatomic location of the anterior segmental bronchus is not readily accessible via the anterior pulmonary hilum because the segmental vasculature to the apical segment of the upper lobe is located more superficially. The apical and anterior veins converge to form the upper trunk of the superior pulmonary vein. The anterior segmental vein is the more inferior and deeply located of the two vessels. Beneath the apical segmental vein branch, the superior trunk of the right pulmonary artery is dissected peripherally, exposing the apical and anterior segmental arterial branches. The more inferiorly located anterior branch is isolated and divided. The interlobar pulmonary vein is gently reflected inferiorly, and the anterior segmental arterial stump and apical segmental vein are reflected superiorly to expose the anterior segmental bronchus. Small venous tributaries often are encountered leading to the interlobar upper lobe vein and must be individually ligated and divided.

Left upper division. An upper-division segmentectomy of the left upper lobe is sometimes referred to as a "lingular sparing" left upper lobectomy. The pleural lining over the upper lobe vein is incised, and the bifurcation between the superior branch of the upper lobe vein and the lingular vein is identified. The superior branch of the upper lobe vein is encircled and transected with the 2.5-mm load of the endostapler. The pulmonary arterial branches to the anterior segment and apical segment of the upper lobe are identified along the superior arch of the pulmonary artery and usually can be isolated with minimal dissection unless peribronchial lymphadenopathy is present. These vessels also may originate as a common trunk. After division of these vessels with the 2.5-mm load of the endostapler, the upper division bronchus can be palpated and bluntly dissected. If necessary, the upper aspect of the major fissure is completed with endostapler application to separate the posterior segment of the upper lobe from the superior segment of the lower lobe. This separation will enhance exposure of the posterior segmental arterial supply, which can be multiple.

The arterial anatomy to the left upper lobe is the most variable of all lobes of the lungs. Attention to this detail can avoid inadvertent injury to segmental vessels that remain intact by a surgeon who incorrectly perceives the dissection to be complete. When dissecting about the superior aspect of the left pulmonary hilum, it also is important to stay within the perivascular plane to avoid possible injury to the left recurrent laryngeal nerve located beneath the aortic arch in the aorticopulmonary window.

Lingulectomy. During lingulectomy, the mediastinal pleural lining is incised along the anterior left hilum. The lingular vein is identified as the lower tributary of the upper lobe pulmonary vein. The lingular bronchus then can be palpated beneath the stump of the lingular vein, and anterior blunt dissection can establish the bifurcation with the upper division bronchus of the upper lobe. Dissection along the inferior aspect of the anterior pulmonary hilum also can establish the division between the lower aspect of the upper lobe vein and the lower lobe venous trunk. Appreciation of this anatomic relationship is important as one proceeds to division of the parenchymal bridge of lung tissue that may exist between the inferior lingular segment and the basilar segments of the lower lobe. This parenchymal bridge is divided using the endostapler to identify the basilar segmental artery posteriorly and the lingular segmental pulmonary artery anteriorly at the interlobar zone of the pulmonary hilum. The interlobar pulmonary artery then is exposed. There may be more than one lingular arterial branch, and these branches must be divided, taking care to avoid inadvertent ligation of the more superiorly located posterior segmental pulmonary artery or arteries. The lingular bronchus is divided without encroachment on the airway to the upper division.

Middle lobectomy/segmentectomy. The right middle lobe has many anatomic and functional similarities to the lingula on the left. The right middle lobe is much smaller than all other regions designated as lobe and presents analogous anatomic and surgical considerations when compared with lingulectomy. It is comprised of two classical anatomic segments, frequently is associated with an incomplete fissure, has venous drainage typically associated with the superior pulmonary vein, and has a discrete arterial branch arising from the main pulmonary artery. Although lateral segmentectomy of the middle lobe can be performed, the authors generally prefer to resect the entire lobe in the management of stage I NSCLC.

After the mediastinal pleura is incised, the right middle lobe vein is identified, which usually arises as the inferior branch from the right superior pulmonary vein. The middle lobe vein can arise as a natural variant from the right inferior pulmonary vein. Therefore the venous anatomy must be delineated carefully before middle lobe vein division. The middle lobe artery (which may be paired) then can be appreciated overlying the middle lobe bronchus, and each is then taken in succession, taking care to preserve the basilar artery and bronchus.

Superior segmentectomy. The approach to superior segmentectomy begins with identification of the interlobar pulmonary artery in the major fissure. Posterior dissection along the course of the interlobar artery will identify the superior segmental artery inferiorly. On the right, a lateral segmental branch of right middle lobe artery usually will be seen medially and proximal to the origin of the superior segmental artery. The posterior segmental artery can be identified slightly proximal and opposite the superior segmental artery on the axis of the interlobar pulmonary artery. Occasionally, the posterior segmental artery will arise from the superior segmental artery. It obviously is important to ligate distal to the posterior segmental vessel artery at this common trunk. The superior segmental bronchus that lies just posterior to the artery is isolated and divided.

When approaching the left lower lobe superior segment, the anatomic relationships are somewhat different. The superior segmental artery is identified posteriorly along the axis of the interlobar artery opposite the more anterior position of the posterior segmental artery branch of the left upper lobe. The relationship of the superior segmental bronchus to the superior segmental artery is similar bilaterally. The superior segmental bronchus can be palpated and visualized with minimal dissection deep to the transected superior segmental arterial stump.

Basilar segmentectomy. Basilar segmentectomy is the resection of all four basilar segments of the lower lobe as a single unit. In many respects, the dissection for a basilar segmentectomy is the mirror image of the dissection for superior segmentectomy. The key issue in performing a basilar segmentectomy is the identification and preservation of the superior segmental vein during the dissection of the basilar segmental vein. The first maneuver is to divide the inferior pulmonary ligament to delineate the inferior aspect of the pulmonary hilum and the detail of the inferior pulmonary vein. The basilar segmental vein usually is a large trunk with a primary bifurcation between it and the superior segmental vein. The parenchymal bridge of the lower aspect of the major fissure between middle lobe on the right or the lingular segment of the upper lobe on the left and the basilar segments of either lobe is divided with the endostapler. This division exposes the basilar segmental artery in the interlobar hilar plane. The middle lobe artery and lingular segmental artery (depending on the side of resection) are identified proximal and anterior to the main basilar arterial trunk. The superior segmental artery of either lower lobe usually is noted proximal and posterior along the course of the interlobar artery as it is dissected from the lower aspect of the main basilar arterial trunk.

At completion of the sublobar resection, the pulmonary specimen is removed from the chest in a specimen retrieval bag, commercially available from a number of endosurgical companies, to avoid contaminating the chest wall by a potentially malignant lesion within the specimen. Alternatively, a sterile operating room latex glove can be introduced into the chest through an intercostal access site to be used as a retrieval bag. Following removal of the specimen, the lung is partially expanded, and the resection staple-line margin is re-examined for hemostasis and air-leak control. A single chest tube is inserted through one of the lower intercostal access sites and is positioned under thoracoscopic guidance toward a posterior apical position. The other intercostal access sites are closed primarily. The chest tube is removed when drainage is minimal and the air leak has resolved customarily on the second or third postoperative day.

Perioperative outcomes

The perioperative outcomes of anatomic segmentectomy can be comparable or superior to those of lobectomy (Table 1) [39]. In the University of Pittsburgh Medical Center series of 182 consecutive segmentectomies, the average operative time was 147 minutes (median, 138 minutes; range, 32–367 minutes) and estimated blood loss was 171 cm^3 (median, 125 cm^3), which was significantly less than that of lobectomy (see Table 1). There were two perioperative deaths (1.1%) subsequent to segmentectomy, both with an open approach. Median hospital stay was 6 days (range, 2–35 days). There were no significant differences in median length of stay or overall rates of complications or mortality between segmentectomy and lobectomy (see Table 1). Complications occurred in 59 segmentectomy patients (32.4%), as outlined in Table 2. The most common complication was atrial fibrillation, which occurred in 17 patients (9.2%). Prolonged air leak (> 5 days) was encountered in 13 patients (7.1%). There was no significant difference between segmentectomy and lobectomy in the overall rates of complications (32.4% versus 33.7%) or of major complications (13.2% versus 13.8%) [39].

Table 1
Comparison of perioperative outcomes of segmentectomy versus lobectomy

	Segmentectomy (n = 182)	Lobectomy (n = 246)	*P*-value
Operative time (min)	147	216	< .001
Estimated blood loss (cm^3)	185	291	< .001
Length of stay (median)	6	6	.2
Complications			
Overall	59 (32.4%)	83 (33.7%)	.43
Major	24 (13.2%)	34 (13.8%)	.48
30-Day mortality	2 (1.1%)	8 (3.3%)	.13

Data from Schuchert MJ, Pettiford BL, Keeley S, et al. Anatomic segmentectomy in the treatment of stage I non-small cell lung cancer. Ann Thorac Surg 2007;84:926–33.

The early results of the American College of Surgeons Oncology Group (ACOSOG) Z0030 trial provides important information on the modern day mortality and morbidity associated with anatomic lung resection for NSCLC, including anatomic segmentectomy [41]. The mortality rate (1.1%) and complication rate (32%) of the University of Pittsburgh experience are comparable to those of Z0030 for segmentectomy (3% and 46%, respectively).

Recurrence and survival

Segmentectomy historically has been associated with increased local recurrence rates. As discussed previously, the LCSG conducted the

Table 2
Complications after anatomic segmentectomy

Complication	Number (%)
Overall	59 (32.4)
Major	24 (13.2)
Complication types	
Cardiac	23 (12.6)
Atrial fibrillation	17
Cardiac arrest	2
Myocardial infarction	1
Congestive heart failure	1
Ventricular arrhythmia	1
Heart block	1
Pulmonary	27 (14.8)
Air leak	13 (7.1)
Pneumonia	9 (4.9)
Bronchoscopy	8
Pneumothorax	7
Re-intubation	6
Tracheostomy	4
Empyema	2
Effusion/drainage	2
Bronchopleural fistula	1
Infectious	16 (8.8)
Pneumonia	9 (4.9)
Empyema	2
Clostridium difficile	1
Wound infection	1
Septicemia	0
Other	
Pulmonary embolism	2
Acute renal failure	2
Delirium	2
Cerebrovascular accident	1
Bleeding/re-operation	1
Deep vein thrombosis	1
Stroke	1

Data from Schuchert MJ, Pettiford BL, Keeley S, et al. Anatomic segmentectomy in the treatment of stage I non-small cell lung cancer. Ann Thorac Surg 2007;84:926–33.

only randomized study comparing sublobar resection with lobectomy in patients who had stage IA NSCLC [11]. The principal finding in this study was a threefold increase in local recurrence (17.2% versus 6.4%) in patients who had sublobar resection, with a 2.4-fold increase in those who had segmental resection. Such studies have established lobectomy as the reference standard in patients who have early-stage lung cancer.

The increased identification of small NSCLC tumors by enhanced CT screening protocols in higher-risk surgical patients [13], however, has led many surgeons to question the appropriateness of lobectomy for these tumors [14,15]. Okada and co-workers [42] compared the results of extended segmentectomy and lobectomy in patients who had T1N0 tumors. The 5-year survival rate of 87.1% among the segmentectomy patients compared quite favorably with the 87.7% survival rate in the lobectomy group. Kondo and associates [43] analyzed the outcomes of 104 patients undergoing resection for peripheral stage IA adenocarcinomas, with particular attention to patients who had lesions smaller than 1 cm in diameter (n = 57). Within this group, 23 lobectomies, 13 segmentectomies, and 21 wedge resections were performed. There was no difference in cancer-free survival regardless of the mode of resection, with an overall 5-year survival rate of 97%. Bando and colleagues [44] similarly reported on a series of 74 patients who had T1N0 NSCLC and noted locoregional recurrence in only 1.9% of the patients who had tumors of 2 cm or less.

In the University of Pittsburgh experience, there were 32 recurrences (17.6%) during the follow-up period—14 locoregional and 18 distant. Mean time to recurrence was 14.3 months. Overall recurrence rates were similar between the segmentectomy (17.6%) and lobectomy (16.7%) groups. The majority of recurrences were seen in patients who had stage IB disease (20/73, 27.4%, versus 12/109, 11.0%, for patients who had stage 1A disease; $P = .004$). There was no difference between segmentectomy and lobectomy in recurrence-free or overall survival [32,39].

In appropriately chosen cases, segmentectomy seems to be associated with no significant difference in recurrence-free or overall survival, especially in patients who have stage IA disease in which adequate margins are achievable. Local recurrence rates may be improved further by the use of local radiation along the surgical margins (brachytherapy), thus augmenting the results of sublobar resection.

Intraoperative brachytherapy

Intraoperative brachytherapy has been proposed as an adjunctive local-control measure following lung resection associated with close or positive margins of resection. This use of adjuvant intraoperative brachytherapy has been employed primarily in the setting of locally advanced lung cancer where margins cannot be achieved reliably and in an effort to provide immediate potential salvage therapy after thoracotomy [45]. D'Amato and colleagues [46] were the first to report the use of intraoperative Iodine-125 (^{125}I) brachytherapy as a local measure following sublobar resection of peripheral stage I lung cancers when pathologically clear surgical margins had been obtained. This approach uses ^{125}I pellets incorporated at 1-cm intervals into a polyglycolate (Vicryl) mesh to create a treatment grid with pellets at 1-cm^2 intervals (Fig. 3A, B). This mesh template then is introduced into the chest and sutured onto the lung parenchymal surface at the suture line of resection to provide at least 2 cm of lateral margin coverage from the resection staple line. Usually 40 to 60 ^{125}I pellets within four to five lines of suture material are used with each brachytherapy implant. The total delivered radiation dose to the local tissues was calculated to be 10,000 cGY at a 1-cm depth. In essence, this very high-intensity local therapy effectively extends the margin of resection by another centimeter. Santos and colleagues [47] subsequently reported the longitudinal follow-up of the use of intraoperative ^{125}I brachytherapy and found that local recurrence following sublobar resection seemed to be significantly reduced compared with historical sublobar resection control cases. This study also revealed that the use of brachytherapy mesh implants was associated with no locally important radiation fibrosis, implant migration, or unexpected decline in postoperative pulmonary function. In addition, the use of radioactive brachytherapy implants has been found to be safe, with minimal radiation exposure to physicians and nursing staff [48].

Other retrospective reports of the use of intraoperative ^{125}I brachytherapy implants used in the setting of sublobar resection have yielded encouraging results. Fernando and associates [18] performed a retrospective multicenter analysis of 291 patients that compared outcomes after lobectomy (n = 167) with outcomes following sublobar resection (n = 124). Nearly one half of the sublobar resection group (n = 60) received adjuvant ^{125}I brachytherapy. The local recurrence rate in the sublobar resection group was decreased from 17.2% to 3.3% with the use of adjuvant ^{125}I brachytherapy. Finally Birdas and colleagues [49] analyzed the outcomes of sublobar resection with brachytherapy for patients who had pathologic stage IB NSCLC. A total of 167 patients who had stage IB disease (126 patients undergoing lobectomy and 41 patients undergoing sublobar resection) were evaluated for local recurrence, disease-free survival, and overall survival. The rate of local recurrence in the sublobar resection with ^{125}I brachytherapy group (4.8%) was similar to that in the lobectomy group (3.2%). There was no statistically significant difference between the two groups in disease-free survival and overall survival. These investigators concluded that sublobar resection with intraoperative ^{125}I brachytherapy provided equivalent local control, disease-free, and overall survival outcomes similar to those for lobectomy in patients who had stage IB NSCLC. They emphasized the potential utility of intraoperative ^{125}I brachytherapy in theoretically "extending" the margin of resection when larger (T2) tumors are chosen for sublobar resection. The efficacy of brachytherapy mesh implantation is being analyzed in a prospective, randomized, multi-institutional trail (ACOSOG Z0432) comparing segmentectomy alone versus segmentectomy with brachytherapy mesh in the setting of stage I NSCLC.

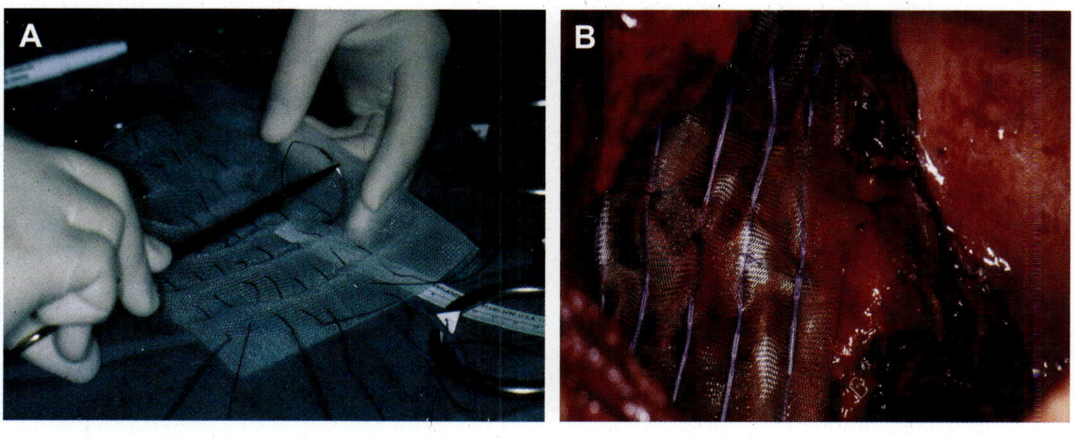

Fig. 3. (*A*) Fabrication of a ^{125}I Vicryl mesh implant. (*B*) The brachytherapy mesh is centered along the margin of resection and is secured with interrupted sutures.

Impact of tumor size and surgical margin

Okada and co-workers [33] evaluated the effect of tumor size on prognosis after resection of 1272 patients. There was no statistical difference in the 5-year disease-free survival in patients who had tumors 2 cm or larger in diameter when treated with lobectomy or segmentectomy (87.4% versus 84.6%, respectively). In another study by Fernando and co-authors [18], lobar and sublobar resection was compared in patients who had T1 tumors. There was no difference in survival in patients undergoing lobar or sublobar resection for tumors smaller than 2 cm, but survival was significantly improved in the lobar group in patients who had tumors 2 to 3 cm in size. Iwasaki and associates [50] performed a case-matched analysis of 86 patients who underwent left upper division segmentectomy versus lobectomy for tumors smaller than 2 cm. There was no difference in morbidity, mortality, recurrence, or survival. The 5-year survival for the segmentectomy group was 69.7%, versus 72.5% for the lobectomy group. Other reports examining sublobar resection in the setting of subcentimeter tumors document no difference in local recurrence or survival [51–53]. These data support the evolving concept that anatomic sublobar resection (anatomic segmentectomy) can be performed with expected survival similar to those of lobectomy in select patients who have small peripheral tumors (in particular those $<$ 2 cm). A prospective, randomized, multi-institutional study (Cancer and Leukemia Group B [CALGB]/Altorki) is underway evaluating the outcomes of sublobar resection compared with lobectomy for early-stage lung cancer (tumors $\leq$ 2 cm).

What constitutes an adequate margin in the setting of segmentectomy remains unresolved. A negative microscopic margin in combination with negative marginal cytology has been suggested to be a reasonable intraoperative approach at margin assessment [54]. Previous recommendations have implied that 1-cm margins might suffice [55]. The concept of an adequate surgical margin is based on the need to clear microscopic alterations in tumor geometry with associated local microscopic extension. In a pathologic analysis of 70 NSCLC surgical resection specimens, the degree of microscopic tumor extension varied based on tumor histology (Fig. 4). These data revealed that to account for 95% of observed microscopic tumor extension, at least a 6-mm margin is necessary in squamous cell carcinoma and an 8-mm

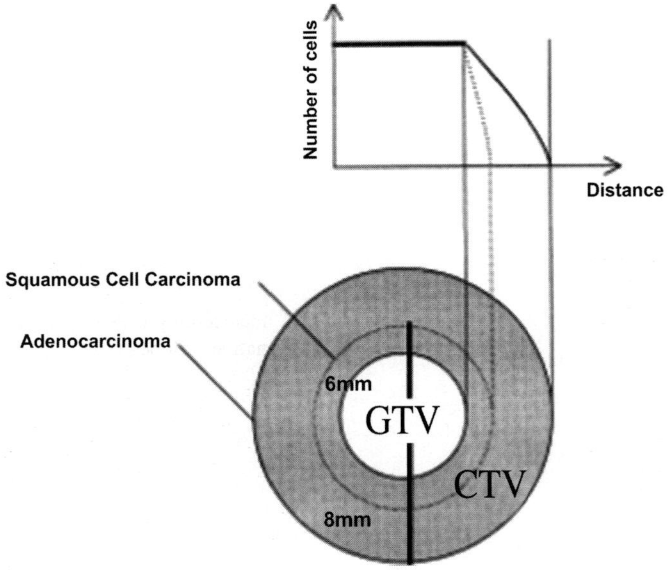

Fig. 4. The impact of microscopic tumor extension on surgical margins encountered in the setting of non-small cell carcinoma. The final recommended clinical target volume (CTV) varies with the histologic subtype of the tumor. Minimum margins to account for 95% of microscopic tumor extension are 8 mm in the setting of adenocarcinoma, compared with 6 mm for squamous cell carcinoma. GTV, gross tumor volume. (*Adapted from* Giraud P, Antoine M, Larrouy A, et al. Evaluation of microscopic tumor extension in non-small cell lung cancer for three dimensional conformal radiotherapy planning. Int J Radiat Oncol Biol Phys 2000;48(4):1023; with permission.)

margin is needed in adenocarcinoma [56]. More recently, Sawabata and colleagues [57] have suggested that to minimize the risk of local recurrence, margin distance should be greater than the maximum diameter of the tumor. El-Sherif and associates [34] analyzed the impact of surgical margin in 87 patients undergoing sublobar resection for stage I NSCLC. Tumor margins of 1 cm or larger were associated with a significantly lower recurrence rate than margins smaller than 1 cm (8% versus 19%; $P = .003$). In the University of Pittsburgh Medical Center experience, a margin-to-tumor ratio of less than 1 was associated with a significant increase in recurrence rates compared with ratios of 1 or larger (25.0% versus 6.2%; $P = .0014$) [39].

Summary

Although lobectomy should continue to be regarded as the procedure of choice for NSCLC, certain subsets of patients who have favorable characteristics may be treated appropriately with segmentectomy without adversely affecting oncologic outcome as long as an adequate assessment of intraoperative nodal status and surgical margin is performed. The use of anatomic segmentectomy may be particularly useful for small, peripheral tumors less than 2 cm in diameter located within anatomic segmental boundaries, as well as for elderly patients who have impaired cardiopulmonary function. Ground-glass opacities and lesions displaying bronchoalveolar histology also may be appropriate target lesions for segmentectomy because of their low metastatic potential. Prospective, randomized studies (such as the CALGB/Altorki trial and the brachytherapy mesh trial) will be necessary to delineate fully the utility of segmentectomy in patients who have NSCLC.

References

[1] Churchill ED, Belsey R. Segmental pneumonectomy in bronchiectasis. Ann Surg 1939;109:481.

[2] Kent EM, Blades B. The anatomic approach to pulmonary resection. Ann Surg 1942;116:782–4.

[3] Overholt RH, Langer L. A new technique for pulmonary segmental resection, its application in the treatment of bronchiectasis. Surg Gynecol Obstet 1947;84:257.

[4] Oschner A, DeBakey M. Primary pulmonary malignancy: treatment by total pneumonectomy. Analysis of 79 collected cases and presentation of 7 personal cases. Surg Gynecol Obstet 1939;68:435–41.

[5] Churchill ED, Sweet RH, Sutter L, et al. The surgical management of carcinoma of the lung. A study of cases treated at the Massachusetts General Hospital from 1930–50. J Thorac Cardiovasc Surg 1950;20:349–65.

[6] Churchill ED, Sweet RH, Scannell JG, et al. Further studies in the surgical management of carcinoma of the lung. J Thorac Surg 1958;36:301–8.

[7] Bonfils-Roberts EA, Claggett OT. Contemporary indication for pulmonary segmental resections. J Thorac Surg 1972;63:433–8.

[8] Jensik RJ, Faber LP, Milloy FJ, et al. Segmental resection for lung cancer—a fifteen year experience. J Thorac Cardiovasc Surg 1973;66:563–72.

[9] Read RC, Yoder G, Schaeffer RC. Survival after conservative resection for TIN0M0 non-small cell lung cancer. Ann Thorac Surg 1990;49:242–7.

[10] Warren WH, Faber LP. Segmentectomy versus lobectomy in patients with stage I pulmonary carcinoma. Five-year survival and patterns of intrathoracic recurrence. J Thorac Cardiovasc Surg 1994;107(4):1087–93.

[11] Ginsburg RJ, Rubenstein LV. Randomized trial of lobectomy versus limited resection for T1N0 non-small cell lung cancer. Ann Thorac Surg 1995;60:615–23.

[12] Landreneau RJ, Sugarbaker DJ, Mack MJ, et al. Wedge resection versus lobectomy for stage I (T1N0M0) non-small cell lung cancer. J Thorac Cardiovasc Surg 1997;113:691–700.

[13] Henschke CI, I-ELCAP Investigators. CT screening for lung cancer: update. Surg Oncol Clin N Am 2005;14(4):761–76.

[14] Lewis RJ. The role of video assisted thoracic surgery for carcinoma of the lung: wedge resection to lobectomy by simultaneous individual stapling. Ann Thorac Surg 1993;56:762–8.

[15] Tang AW, Moss HA, Robertson RJ. The solitary pulmonary nodule. Eur J Radiol 2003;45(1):69–77.

[16] Rehders A, Hosch SB, Scheunemann P, et al. Benefit of surgical treatment of lung metastasis in soft tissue sarcoma. Arch Surg 2007;142:70–5.

[17] Okada M, Yoshikawa K, Hatta T, et al. Is segmentectomy with lymph node assessment an alternative to lobectomy for non-small cell lung cancer of 2 cm or smaller? Ann Thorac Surg 2001;71:956–61.

[18] Fernando HC, Santos R, Benfield JR, et al. Lobar and sublobar resection with and without brachytherapy for small stage IA non-small cell lung cancer. J Thorac Cardiovasc Surg 2005;129(2):261–7.

[19] Pettiford BL, Schuchert MJ, Santos R, et al. Role of sublobar resection (segmentectomy and wedge resection) in the surgical management of non-small cell lung cancer. Thorac Surg Clin 2007;17(2):175–90.

[20] Pennathur A, Abbas G, Christie N, et al. Video-assisted thoracoscopic surgery and lobectomy, sublobar resection, radiofrequency ablation, and stereotactic radiosurgery: advances and controversies in the

management of early-stage non-small cell lung cancer. Curr Opin Pulm Med 2007;13(4):267–70.

[21] Yoshida J, Nagai K, Yokose T, et al. Limited resection trial for pulmonary ground-glass opacity nodules; Fifty case experience. J Thorac Cardiovasc Surg 2005;129:991–6.

[22] Ginsberg RJ, Hill LD, Eagen RT, et al. Modern thirty day operative mortality for surgical resections in lung cancer. J Thorac Cardiovasc Surg 1983;86: 654–8.

[23] Wada H, Nakamura T, Nakamoto K, et al. Thirty day operative mortality for thoracotomy in lung cancer. J Thorac Cardiovasc Surg 1998;115:70–3.

[24] Keenan RJ, Landreneau RJ, Maley RH Jr, et al. Segmental resection spares pulmonary function in patients with stage I lung cancer. Ann Thorac Surg 2004;78:228–33.

[25] Harada H, Okada M, Sakamoto T, et al. Functional advantage after radical segmentectomy versus lobectomy for lung cancer. Ann Thorac Surg 2005;80: 2041–5.

[26] Silvestri GA, Gould MK, Margolis ML, et al. American College of Chest Physicians. Noninvasive staging of non-small cell lung cancer: ACCP evidenced-based clinical practice guidelines (2nd edition). Chest 2007;132(3 Suppl):178S–201S.

[27] Detterbeck FC, Jantz MA, Wallace M, et al. American College of Chest Physicians. Invasive mediastinal staging of lung cancer: ACCP evidence-based clinical practice guidelines (2nd edition). Chest 2007;132(3 Suppl):202S–20S.

[28] Rankin SC. Staging of non-small cell lung cancer (NSCLC). Cancer Imaging 2006;6:1–3.

[29] Erturan S, Yaman M, Aydin G, et al. The role of whole-body bone scanning and clinical factors in detecting bone metastases in patients with non-small cell lung cancer. Chest 2005;127(2):449–54.

[30] Schuchert MJ, Luketich JD, Fernando HC. Video-assisted thoracic surgery. In: Norton JA, Barie BS, Bollinger RR, et al, editors. Surgery: basic science and clinical evidence. 2nd edition. New York: Springer-Verlag, in press.

[31] Colice GL, Shafazand S, Griffin JP, et al. American College of Chest Physicians. Physiologic evaluation of the patient with lung cancer being considered for resectional surgery: ACCP evidence-based clinical practice guidelines (2nd edition). Chest 2007; 132(3 Suppl):161S–77S.

[32] El-Sherif A, Gooding WE, Santos R, et al. Outcomes of sublobar resection versus lobectomy for stage I non-small cell lung cancer: a 13-year analysis. Ann Thorac Surg 2006;82:408–16.

[33] Okada M, Nishio M, Sakamoto T, et al. Effect of tumor size on prognosis in patients with non-small cell lung cancer: the role of segmentectomy as a type of lesser resection. J Thorac Cardiovasc Surg 2005; 129(1):87–93.

[34] El-sherif A, Fernando HC, Santos R, et al. Margin and local recurrence after sublobar resection of non-small cell lung cancer. Ann Surg Oncol 2007; 14(8):2400–5.

[35] Landreneau RJ, Hazelrigg SR, Mack MJ, et al. Postoperative pain-related morbidity: video-assisted thoracic surgery versus thoracotomy. Ann Thorac Surg 1993;56(6):1285–9.

[36] Nagahiro I, Andou A, Aoe M, et al. Pulmonary function, postoperative pain, and serum cytokine level after lobectomy: a comparison of VATS and conventional procedure. Ann Thorac Surg 2001; 72(2):362–5.

[37] Tschernko EM, Hofer S, Bieglmayer C, et al. Early postoperative stress: video-assisted wedge resection/lobectomy vs. conventional axillary thoracotomy. Chest 1996;109(6):1636–42.

[38] Demmy TL, Curtis JJ. Minimally invasive lobectomy directed toward frail and high-risk patients: a case-control study. Ann Thorac Surg 1999;68(1): 194–200.

[39] Schuchert MJ, Pettiford BL, Keeley S, et al. Anatomic segmentectomy in the treatment of stage I non-small cell lung cancer. Ann Thorac Surg 2007; 84:926–33.

[40] Nakamura H, Kazuyuki S, Kawasaki N, et al. History of limited resection for non-small cell lung cancer. Ann Thorac Cardiovasc Surg 2005;11(6): 356–62.

[41] Allen MS, Darling GE, Pechet TTV, et al. Morbidity and mortality of major pulmonary resections in patients with early-stage lung cancer: initial results of the randomized, prospective ACOSOG Z0030 trial. Ann Thorac Surg 2006;81:1013–20.

[42] Okada M, Sakamoto T, Nishio W, et al. Characteristics and prognosis of patients after resection of non-small cell lung carcinoma measuring 2 cm or less in greatest dimension. Cancer 2003;988:535–41.

[43] Kondo D, Yamada K, Kitayama Y, et al. Peripheral lung adenocarcinomas: 10mm or less in diameter. Ann Thorac Surg 2003;76:350–5.

[44] Bando T, Yamigahara K, Kitayama G, et al. A new method of segmental resection for primary lung cancer: intermediate results. Eur J Cardiothorac Surg 2002;21:894–9.

[45] Nori D, Li X, Pugkhem T. Intraoperative brachytherapy using Gelfoam radioactive implants for resected stage III non-small cell lung cancer with positive margin: a pilot study. J Surg Oncol 1995;4: 257–61.

[46] D'Amato TA, Galloway M, Szydlowski G, et al. Intraoperative brachytherapy following thoracoscopic wedge resection of stage I lung cancer. Chest 1998;114:1112–5.

[47] Santos R, Colonias A, Parda D, et al. Comparison between sublobar resection and 125Iodine brachytherapy after sublobar resection in high-risk patients with stage I non-small-cell lung cancer. Surgery 2003;134:691–7.

[48] Smith RP, Schuchert MJ, Komanduri K, et al. Dosimetric evaluation of radiation exposure during

^{125}I Vicryl mesh implants: implications for ACOSOG Z4032. Ann Surg Oncol 2007;14:3610–3.

[49] Birdas TJ, Koehler RP, Colonias A, et al. Sublobar resection with brachytherapy versus lobectomy for stage IB non-small cell lung cancer. Ann Thorac Surg 2006;81(2):434–8.

[50] Iwasaki A, Hamanaka W, Hamada T, et al. Comparison between a case-matched analysis of left upper lobe trisegmentectomy and left upper lobectomy for small size lung cancer located in the upper division. Thorac Cardiovasc Surg 2007;55(7):454–7.

[51] Martin-Ucar AE, Nakas A, Pilling JE, et al. A case-matched study of anatomical segmentectomy versus lobectomy for stage I lung cancer in high-risk patients. Eur J Cardiothorac Surg 2005;27:675–9.

[52] Ketchedjian A, Daly B, Landreneau R, et al. Sublobar resection for the subcentimeter pulmonary nodule. Semin Thorac Cardiovasc Surg 2005;17(2):128–33.

[53] Okada M, Koike T, Higashiyama M, et al. Radical sublobar resection for small-sized non-small cell lung cancer: a multicenter study. J Thorac Cardiovasc Surg 2006;132:769–75.

[54] Higashiyama M, Kodama K, Takami K. Intraoperative lavage cytologic analysis of surgical margins in patients undergoing limited surgery for lung cancer. J Thorac Cardiovasc Surg 2003;125:101–7.

[55] Allen MS, Pairolero PC. Inadequacy, mortality and thoracoscopy. Ann Thorac Surg 1995;59:6.

[56] Giraud P, Antoine M, Larrouy A, et al. Evaluation of microscopic tumor extension in non-small cell lung cancer for three dimensional conformal radiotherapy planning. Int J Radiat Oncol Biol Phys 2000;48(4):1015–24.

[57] Sawabata N, Ohta M, Nagakawa K. Optimal distance of malignant negative margin excision of non-small cell lung cancer: a multicenter prospective study. Ann Thorac Surg 2004;77(2):415–20.

ELSEVIER
SAUNDERS

Thorac Surg Clin 18 (2008) 107–112

THORACIC
SURGERY
CLINICS

The Use of Scoring Systems in Selecting Patients for Lung Resection: Work-up Bias Comes Full-Circle

Martin Utley, PhD, Tom Treasure, MD, FRCS*

Clinical Operational Research Unit, University College London, Gower Street, WC1E 6BT, London, UK

The process of selecting patients for lung resection is complex and, to outsiders such as the first author, fascinating. There are many good, clear accounts of the individual roles of different forms of clinical information (radiographs, CT, PET, pathology, or spirometry) in determining diagnosis, TNM stage, and the other important factors that determine the choice of treatment. Less is written about the process by which management decisions emerge from a clinical team. The team must balance, negotiate, or choose from a wealth of internal and external inputs including patient-specific data, published evidence, national guidelines, local protocols, and the experience, opinion, and preferences of a number of health care professionals, not forgetting the wishes of the patient.

In an ideal world one might consider all the information available, sort it into some order of importance to the case under discussion, and then agree on diagnosis, stage, and management plan. That is not quite how the process works in practice. In the authors' observations of many multidisciplinary meetings, experienced chest physicians, surgeons, oncologists, radiologists, and pathologists assimilate these streams of independent evidence and do indeed agree on the most likely histology, the most likely stage of the disease, and the fitness of the patient for treatment. The negotiation of the agreed diagnosis and stage, however, has started before and continues during each specialty's presentation of its findings rather than being held until all the information is set out. It is perhaps natural that people do not wish the findings from their specialty, be it CT, PET, or pathology, to be at odds with the majority view. As an example, in a recent lung cancer multidisciplinary meeting, a pathologist was equivocal as to whether the sample from a solitary pulmonary nodule confirmed a diagnosis of primary lung cancer. Further discussion of the patient elicited a statement as to the patient's smoking history, at which point the pathologist exclaimed, "Well if you'd told me that ..." So much for the independence of the reported findings from each specialty, despite the independence of the raw information available. To a scientist coming from outside a medical background, this experience revealed how information that might seem to be incontrovertible can be renegotiated during the decision-making process.

It is into this melting pot that information based on surgical-risk scoring systems can be added. Perhaps because risk models are constructed using valid statistical techniques, often are based on objective measurements, and often give estimates of risk to several decimal places, there can be a tendency to place excessive trust in the estimates obtained. This article discusses some of the limitations of scoring systems of perioperative risk or longer-term survival that should be kept in mind, particularly in terms of their role in guiding the selection of patients for surgery. Before discussing these limitations, it is worth revisiting briefly the purpose of selection.

The purpose of selecting patients for surgery

Surgeons judge themselves and are judged by others according to the levels of perioperative mortality and morbidity among their patients and the duration and quality of postoperative survival.

* Corresponding author.
E-mail address: tom.treasure@gmail.com
(T. Treasure).

1547-4127/08/$ - see front matter
doi:10.1016/j.thorsurg.2007.10.005

thoracic.theclinics.com

During the workings of the multidisciplinary team and in discussions with patients, selection of patients appropriate for surgery, balancing the short-term risks against long-term survival, is a key contribution of the surgeon.

The original use of scoring systems in cardiothoracic surgery was to redress the imbalance caused by differential selection of cases between the private and the university systems in the United States when coronary artery surgery was burgeoning. There was a perception that the private clinics could "cherry pick" low-risk cases, leaving the higher-risk patients (those who were older, hypertensive, diabetic, or had damaged ventricles) to the university hospitals. The proposed system made it "feasible to analyze operative results by risk groups and to compare results in similar groups between institutions" [1]. In coronary artery surgery, the determinants of long-term outcome (the completeness of restoration of coronary blood flow and the maintenance of myocardial function) also are the predominant factors determining perioperative survival rates. In cancer surgery, however, strategies to reduce risk in the short term may run counter to the long-term benefit of eradication of the cancer. Using low perioperative mortality rates as a measure of the system may be counterproductive [2].

At a population level, the objective in selecting patients for surgery is to maximize the net benefit conferred to all patients who have lung cancer by a team deploying a range of treatment modalities. For this reason, although low perioperative mortality rates are, of course, desirable, the prime objective in selecting patients for surgery is not to minimize perioperative mortality rates. Furthermore, although long postoperative survival among surgical cases is, of course, desirable, the objective in selecting patients for surgery is not to maximize postoperative survival among the patients who undergo surgery, because this metric would ignore the fate of patients who do not undergo surgery.

The goal of the process is to achieve the overall best health gain for all lung cancer patients rather than to produce apparently favorable short- or long-term data sets for surgeons and their institutions. Net benefit is some amalgam of the length of survival and the perceived quality of that survival. This factor is difficult enough to define at an individual level, let alone a population level; it is perhaps beyond language, and quantifying it is perhaps beyond science. Nevertheless decisions must be made by clinicians and patients, so an attempt to realize net benefit must be made.

Most would argue that individual patients have the right to be more or to be less risk-averse and to be more or to be less accepting of death or tenacious of life than the statisticians, health economists, and actuaries might recommend. As an aside, this acceptance of individual patient attitudes is not necessarily in conflict with maximizing net benefit among the patient population as a whole; rather, it is more a reflection that the correct amalgam constituting net benefit is potentially different for each person. For surgery, it is finally the surgeon's responsibility to ensure that the patient's decision is an informed one, and the use of models of risk and survival can contribute to this process. Indeed, many consider quantifying the likelihood of different outcomes so that treatment options can be considered in an informed way to be the primary purpose of models of perioperative risk and of long-term survival. In these discussions the chances of surgical cure are balanced implicitly against the risk of operative mortality, the postoperative morbidity, the permanent reduction in lung function associated with major surgery, and the inevitable course of the disease if the primary tumor is not resected. The use of risk and survival models is intended to make that complex trade of pros and cons explicit.

Risk models: what goes in and what comes out

The first task in constructing a model of perioperative risk or postoperative survival is to identify "candidate prognostic factors" and amass data on these factors and the outcomes of interest. More often than not, it is a case of identifying candidate factors from an existing data set. Ideally, candidate factors should be objective measures that are available for all patients and that bear a putative relationship to the outcome to be predicted (for a broader discussion of these points, see [3]).

Data analysis, typically using regression techniques [4] but increasingly based on other techniques such as neural networks (eg, see [5]), is undertaken to identify which of the candidate factors are associated independently with the outcome measure of interest. These factors then are used to derive an equation for the perioperative risk or the postoperative survival curve that applies to any group of patients that have a given presentation in terms of these factors.

Risk scores are clearly of limited use in selecting patients for surgery if they rely on data not available at the time of the decision, such as pathologic stage. At a more subtle level, the inclusion of treatment-related factors, such as the extent of the resection, presents a similar problem. A decision to perform a sublobar resection typically is made only for patients considered unlikely to tolerate a lobectomy; it almost is the result of the selection process rather than a free choice open to surgeon and patient within that process.

A useful review article by Birim and colleagues [6] tabulates the clinical, tumor-, and treatment-related factors recently found to be associated with perioperative mortality and morbidity and those recently found to be associated with long-term survival. Among factors associated with perioperative mortality and morbidity, age was identified in 9 of 17 papers, forced expiratory volume in 1 second (FEV_1) in 7, cardiovascular disease in 5, sex in 3, Charlson comorbidity index in 2, hypertension in 2, and a number of factors, including diffusing capacity of the lung for carbon dioxide (DLCO), pathologic stage, and American Society of Anesthesiologists classification, were identified in a single paper.

Among factors associated with long-term survival, pathologic stage was identified in 12 of 13 papers, histology in 5, age in 5, FEV_1 in 4, sex in 2, smoking in 2, and a number of factors, including chronic obstructive pulmonary disease, hypertension, and creatinine level, were identified in a single paper.

Interpreting models of risk and survival

If numerous studies identify the same clinical factor as being associated with increased risk or poor survival, this agreement strengthens the notion that this identification is a true finding rather than a statistical fluke. If a factor is identified in only one study, this fact could reflect simply that the item of data was collected in only that study. For instance, when constructing a model for the risk of in-hospital death following lung resection, using data from the European Thoracic Database Project [7], the authors had DLCO data available for less than a third of patients and did not have details of Charlson comorbidity index (to give just one example) for any of the 3426 patients included in the study.

None of the 13 studies mentioned in the previous section identified more than four factors as being independently associated with differential survival following lung resection. There are statistical limitations to identifying many prognostic factors because of the number of deaths in the databases. (Statisticians may be heard grumbling that the perioperative mortality rate is too low to allow them to build good models.) Nevertheless, there is a pragmatic limit to the number of data items that can be completed accurately for all cases.

These observations point to an intrinsic limitation in relating risk scores and survival models to individual patients and hence in the use of such modeling to inform decisions concerning surgery. Risk models are not complete. It would be entirely wrong to suppose that a clinical feature does not affect the risk for a particular patient simply because that feature does not appear in a risk model. The feature could be innocuous; it could be a dangerous but rare clinical feature that, because of its rarity is not found to be statistically significant in the model-building exercise; it could be a dangerous (common or otherwise) feature that was not entered into the risk model as a candidate factor through oversight or because this item of data was not recorded in a sufficient proportion of patients; it could be a common feature that is so dangerous, and widely accepted as dangerous, that it is rare among patients selected for surgery. However hard one looks, the risk equation or spreadsheet application does not hold the answer.

The last possibility mentioned in the previous paragraph illustrates a much bigger problem: the flawed logic of using a risk model based on data from patients who were selected for and had surgery to inform decisions about who should be selected for surgery in the future. When presenting the risk model for lung resection, a member of the audience asked why "recent stroke" had not been found to be a risk factor. In response, it was pointed out that, quite apart from the relatively low prevalence of recent stroke among patients presenting with lung cancer, recent stroke is such a clear contraindication to lung resection that no surgeon in his or her right mind would perform surgery in this context. Hence, no patients who had experienced a recent stroke would enter the surgical database used to construct the risk model.

For this reason, factors that preclude surgery are never included in models derived from surgical databases. Unless the use of clinical judgment is outlawed, this omission is, in itself, unlikely to have a damaging impact on the quality of patient selection. There are more subtle effects, however.

Ideally, what one would say to a patient is that, "among people exactly like you the prospects following resection are such and such." All one knows, however, are the prospects following resection among people who had some similar characteristics and who were offered and opted to have surgery.

Suppose a group of surgical candidates had many clinical features in common, to the extent that using an accepted model derived from a surgical database would give the same estimate for the postoperative course for each patient within the group (eg, a 60% chance of surviving to 5 years). Given the incomplete nature of risk models, there will be patient-to-patient differences, evident before operation, which may indicate that some subgroups of patients will do better than others.

Consider the scenario in which some patients do not have surgery for reasons based on adverse clinical factors that were not included in the survival model. It is likely that these clinical judgments are similar to those applied among the patients in the data set from which the model was derived. The patients who do go on to have surgery can be expected to mirror the selected patients in the surgical database from which the survival model emerged. The prediction of 60% survival at 5 years may well be vindicated on subsequent statistical analysis.

Now consider the alternative: despite some patients having adverse clinical factors external to the survival model, the model is followed slavishly, and all the patients undergo surgery. It is reasonable to suppose that 5-year survival within this less selected group would fall below the 60% estimated using the survival model. It follows that the surgeon would not have been correct to quote 60% 5-year survival to the whole patient group, because this estimate fails to account for the some of the adversely predictive clinical factors that excluded patients from the data used to build the model.

Using estimates derived from statistical models without taking due account of the provenance of the data that underpin the model can, in this way, subvert the process of clinical selection. This lapse in judgment can happen when, on the basis of multivariate analysis, exponents of a new intervention present factors associated with good and bad prognosis and advocate the intervention for use among patient groups defined by these factors, forgetting all the other criteria that they used carefully to select the patients on whom to experiment.

One might argue that this problem could be avoided if a risk model was used that incorporated more clinical factors to give a finer categorization of patients, but this argument misses the point. However finely the patient population is stratified in terms of risk, there may always be patient characteristics that contribute, in an explicit or tacit fashion, to the decision to operate, with the effect of selecting out patients thought to be at greater risk or thought to have less to gain. Unless all patients within a particular risk group are operated upon, or unless those that are not operated on opt out of surgery on nonclinical grounds, the estimate of surgical risk applied to a group of patients at the time of the decision to operate is likely to be an underestimate, and the estimate of surgical benefit likely to be an overestimate.

The logical (and some may suggest sophistic) arguments given presented here, which are merely further examples of the phenomenon of work-up bias [8], suggest that one should exercise caution in using risk models to inform decisions to opt for surgery. In one area, however, the construction of risk models can play a definite role: in identifying patients who do not benefit from surgery. If, from multivariate analysis of patients carefully selected for surgery by teams of experienced clinicians, a factor or combination of factors emerges that is clearly associated with unacceptably high short-term risk or unacceptably poor long-term survival, a strong case can be made for no longer operating on the patients who meet these criteria unless, fully informed, the patient is adamant.

The appropriateness of risk models over time

Models of perioperative risk become out of date. Although the language is of "intrinsic risk faced by the patient" and "patient related risk," improvements in surgical and anesthetic techniques (including the adoption of new technology) and the standards of intensive care mean that the risks faced by different groups of patients change over time. This development is widely understood; for example, few cardiac surgeons today boast of "outperforming" the Parsonnet risk-scoring system developed in the late 1980s. (They may, of course, have become less prone to boasting.) Another mechanism whereby risk models may become out of date also applies to models of long-term survival. Suppose that a surgical risk model became widely accepted and used in the selection of patients. Specifically, suppose that a certain category of patients was shown to have poor postoperative survival. What could be expected if another risk model–building exercise was performed 10 years later? It could be that no patients exhibiting the unfavorable characteristics populate the new surgical database; alternatively it could be that there are such patients but that they are considered by clinical teams to be patients for whom the risk model, for one reason or another, was not the whole picture. Either way, if the first risk model changes clinical practice in selecting patients, it is unlikely the same factors will emerge with the same relationship to risk in a later risk model. In short, risk modeling changes patient selection, which changes the characteristics of the surgical population, which inevitably changes the form of risk model that is appropriate. In the absence of clinical common sense and an awareness of the intrinsic limits to the appropriate use of risk scores, one can almost imagine cyclic patterns of risk model and surgical population.

One conclusion does emerge from such considerations: if, repeatedly, over many years, published risk models show the same combination of clinical features to be associated with very poor outcome, this repetition indicates that such patients continue to be operated on, suggesting that little heed is taken of the findings contained within such publications when selecting patients. As one example, early series of pulmonary metastasectomy for colorectal cancer showed that patients who had raised carcinoembryonic antigen (CEA) levels had very poor 5-year survival [9,10]. Later series report a similar proportion of surgical patients with raised prethoracotomy CEA levels and poor 5-year survival [11–15].

Summary

The construction of statistical models of perioperative risk and long-term postoperative survival is a useful activity. It facilitates fair assessment of surgical outcomes and provides insight into the association between certain clinical features and outcome. It provides quantitative estimates of risk or long-term survival. There are, however, a number of limitations to the use of such models in informing decisions concerning the selection of patients for lung resection. In essence, the limitations described in this article are those of work-up bias [8] come full circle. Concerning the use of scoring systems in selecting patients for resection, one should remember the advice of the wise Gene Blackstone: caveat emptor. The findings of model-building exercises, if based on surgical databases, can only augment, and not replace, clinical judgment. When models suggest that certain patient groups do well, the prior selection of these patients should be borne in mind. When models of perioperative risk or long-term survival suggest that certain patient groups, despite being carefully selected by clinical teams, do badly, this information should be heeded. That said, moves to deny informed patients lung resection on the basis of estimates of risk or "poor" survival should be considered carefully. For example the British Thoracic Society Guidelines on Surgery for lung cancer state that mortality following resection should not be in excess of 4% for lobectomy [16]. It is not exactly clear what is intended by publishing that statement. It represents some form of audit standard but clearly fails if one thinks in terms of the individual patient. A patient who has a curable cancer and who faces a life expectancy likely to be under 2 years without surgery might well accept a greater than 1 in 25 chance of perioperative death. If 25 patients in a room were facing that prospect, all 25 might reasonably hope to be among the 24 expected survivors and opt for surgery [17].

References

[1] Parsonnet V, Dean D, Bernstein AD. A method of uniform stratification of risk for evaluating the results of surgery in acquired adult heart disease. Circulation 1989;79:I3–12.

[2] Treasure T, Utley M, Bailey A. Assessment of whether in-hospital mortality for lobectomy is a useful standard for the quality of lung cancer surgery: retrospective study. BMJ 2003;327:73–4.

[3] Treasure T, Utley M, Berrisford R. A risk model for lung resection: data from the European thoracic database project. Eur J Anaesthesiol, in press.

[4] Hosmer DW, Lemeshow S. Applied logistic regression. New York: Wiley; 1989.

[5] Dolgobrodov SG, Moore P, Marshall R, et al. Artificial neural network: predicted vs. observed survival in patients with colonic cancer. Dis Colon Rectum 2007;50:184–91.

[6] Birim O, Kappetein P, van Klaveren R, et al. Prognostic factors in nonsmall cell lung cancer. Eur J Surg Oncol 2006;32:12–23.

[7] Berrisford R, Brunelli A, Rocco G, et al. Audit and guidelines committee of the European Society of Thoracic Surgeons. European Association for Cardio-thoracic Surgery, The European Thoracic

Surgery Database project: modelling the risk of in-hospital death following lung resection. Eur J Cardiothorac Surg 2005;28:306–11.

[8] Blackstone EH, Lauer MS. Caveat emptor: the treachery of work-up bias. J Thorac Cardiovasc Surg 2004;128:341–4.

[9] McAfee MK, Allen MS, Trastek VF, et al. Colorectal lung metastases: results of surgical excision. Ann Thorac Surg 1992;53:780–5.

[10] Girard P, Ducreux M, Baldeyrou P, et al. Surgery for lung metastases from colorectal cancer: analysis of prognostic factors. J Clin Oncol 1996;14: 2047–53.

[11] Zink S, Kayser G, Gabius HJ, et al. Survival, disease-free interval, and associated tumor features in patients with colon/rectal carcinomas and their resected intra-pulmonary metastases. Eur J Cardiothorac Surg 2001;19:908–13.

[12] Rena O, Casadio C, Viano F, et al. Pulmonary resection for metastases from colorectal cancer: factors influencing prognosis. Twenty-year experience. Eur J Cardiothorac Surg 2002;21:906–12.

[13] Higashiyama M, Kodama K, Higaki N, et al. Surgery for pulmonary metastases from colorectal cancer: the importance of prethoracotomy serum carcinoembryonic antigen as an indicator of prognosis. Jpn J Thorac Cardiovasc Surg 2003;51:289–96.

[14] Iizasa T, Suzuki M, Yoshida S, et al. Prediction of prognosis and surgical indications for pulmonary metastasectomy from colorectal cancer. Ann Thorac Surg 2006;82:254–60.

[15] Yedibela S, Klein P, Feuchter K, et al. Surgical management of pulmonary metastases from colorectal cancer in 153 patients. Ann Surg Oncol 2006;13: 1538–44.

[16] British Thoracic Society guidelines on the selection of patients with lung cancer for surgery. Thorax 2001;56:89–108.

[17] Treasure T. Whose lung is it anyway? Thorax 2002; 57:3–4.

ELSEVIER
SAUNDERS

Thorac Surg Clin 18 (2008) 113–118

THORACIC
SURGERY
CLINICS

The Influence of Preoperative Risk Stratification on Fast-Tracking Patients After Pulmonary Resection

Ayesha S. Bryant, MSPH, MD[a,b],
Robert J. Cerfolio, MD, FACS, FCCP[a,*]

[a]Division of Cardiothoracic Surgery, Department of Surgery, University of Alabama at Birmingham, 703 19th Street S, ZRB 739, Birmingham, AL 35294, USA

[b]Department of Epidemiology, University of Alabama at Birmingham School of Public Health, Ryals Public Health Building, 1665 University Boulevard, Birmingham, AL 35294-0022, USA

Concerns about cost effectiveness have changed how physicians have practiced over the past decade. The concepts of hospital costs compared with true cost and how they affect reimbursement from third-party payers and health maintenance organizations have become common themes discussed at national meetings. Although our main goal as physicians and surgeons remains to perform a safe operation, to minimize morbidity and mortality, and to provide the highest quality of our care and satisfaction to our patients, these goals must be accomplished in a cost-conscious setting. The cost of any operation can be divided into several categories: preoperative evaluation, intraoperative costs (equipment, personnel, surgeon fees, anesthesiologist fees, and time in the operating room), and postoperative care. The latter is affected primarily by hospital length of stay, which in patients who undergo pulmonary resection is mainly determined by air leaks, chest tube removal, pain control, or other complications such as arrhythmias. Thus hospital length of stay may be the easiest parameter for the surgeon to unilaterally modify. Patient care protocols help standardize care, minimize the length of the learning curve for fast-tracking, and avoid unnecessary costs [1,2]. This is especially true in a university setting, where there is a constant flux of medical students, residents, and fellows who compose the thoracic team [3]. Fast-tracking protocols allow for the consistent management of the main factors that delay hospital discharge after pulmonary resection, however. These include chest tube management to expedite tube removal, air leak management, and pain control. In addition, the careful review of the results of fact-tracking protocols can help identify select groups of patients who fail fast-tracking. This affords the surgeon the opportunity to modify specific aspects of the fast-track protocols for these select patients. This article attempts to demonstrate that these changes can lead to reduced morbidity and the fast-tracking of even some high-risk patients (Table 1).

Modifiable aspects of postoperative care for the improvement in fast-tracking

Chest tube removal protocols to fast-track patients

One modifiable factor for fast-tracking is the management of chest tubes. Most patients' discharge is contingent on the removal of their chest tubes. Removal of chest tubes is governed primarily by amount of drainage and the presence or absence of air leak. Although much study has been done recently on the problems of air leak, only about 5% to 20% of patients have an air leak on postoperative day 3, when most patients should be able to be discharged. A majority of thoracic surgeons prefer to leave chest tubes in until the air leak has resolved and the output is less than 250 cc/day [4], and some even use 200 cc/day [5]. In a recent poll at a national meeting of general thoracic surgeons, approximately 75%

* Corresponding author.
E-mail address: rcerfolio@uab.edu (R.J. Cerfolio).

doi:10.1016/j.thorsurg.2007.10.002

Table 1
Modifiable (non-patient characteristic) factors that may lead to improved fast-tracking rates

Management	Recommendations
CT management	Most patients can be safely discharged home with up to 450 cc/day drainage.
Air leak management	Discharge home with air leaks on a Heimlich valve type system.
Pain control protocols	Remove thoracic epidural early AM of POD 2 and start oral pain medications.
	Preoperatively identify chronic pain medication users and plan to provide adequate dose postoperatively.
	Intraoperatively use rib- and nerve-sparing techniques.
Social	Assess social support system during preoperative visit. Place orders for home health, rehabilitation, or nursing home placement before surgery to ensure timely delivery.

Abbreviation: POD, postoperative day.

stated they use 250 cc/day as their cutoff value for the removal of chest tubes following lung resection. Thus patient length of stay is often prolonged because of "the drainage being too high." Despite the fact that the patient may otherwise be ready for discharge, the volume of drainage prevents it, even though there are few data to support leaving the patient's tube in. In the authors' recently published series that examined the chest tube removal in 2077 patients [6], 19% of patients were able to go home early on postoperative day (POD) 2, 30% on POD 3, and 15% on POD 4 using the threshold of 450 cc/day instead of the standard 250 cc/day. A total of 364 patients (18%) of the 1988 patients in this series who were sent home without a chest tube thus enjoyed an early hospital discharge [6]. Only 19 of these (5%) were readmitted, and readmission was only secondary to an ipsilateral pleural effusion in a few. This is similar to the readmission rate for the entire patient population, and thus the removal of tubes with a high output does not seem to increase the readmission rate. This provides more evidence that the removal of chest tubes with drainage greater than 250 cc/day but less than 450 cc/day is safe. The authors also observed, however, that patients who spent more time in the hospital (one standard deviation above the average) were more likely to be readmitted, and thus these patients may not be amenable to fast-tracking protocols.

Air leak protocols to fast-track patients

Alveolar-pleural fistulas (air leaks) are a common clinical problem, and remain the most common complication after elective pulmonary resection and video-assisted procedures. Recently, several prospective randomized trials have studied air leaks [7]. An objective, reproducible classification system has been designed, reported, and clinically validated to help study air leaks. This system and these studies have shown that water seal is superior to wall suction to help stop most air leaks [8,9]. The authors have shown that even in patients who have a pneumothorax and an air leak, water seal is safe and best; however, if a patient has a large leak (greater than an expiratory 3 on the classification system) or experiences subcutaneous emphysema or an expanding pneumothorax that causes hypoxia, then some suction (-10 cm of water) should be applied to the chest tubes [10]. This concept of some suction being best for large leaks or leaks that lead to an expanding pneumothorax has been driven home by the work of Brunelli and colleagues. They have presented excellent prospective randomized data that suggest that suction, at least at night, may help seal air leaks by encouraging pleural-pleural apposition, which is a critical component of the healing of air leaks [11,12]. In addition, Brunelli and coworkers [13] have shown that if a pleural tent is performed during upper lobectomy, it may decrease the incidence of an air leak. This is an example of a proactive step that is applied to a select group of patients who are at high risk for complications in an effort to help reduce that complication. Hence the knowledge of risk factors for air leaks can help identify other patients who are at risk for the developing of chronic air leaks.

Patients who have a history of chronic steroid use, of male gender, and those who have a large leak or a leak with a pneumothorax have been shown to be at greater risk for a persistent air leak [14]. Brunelli and colleagues [15] have also shown that a low predicted postoperative forced expiratory volume in 1 second (FEV_1), the presence of pleural adhesions, and an upper or bilobectomy lobectomy are other factors that increase the risk of a persistent air leak. In the authors' experience, patients who had prolonged air leaks scored less than an expiratory 5 on the Robert David Cerfolio (RDC) classification system may be discharged home safely on a Heimlich valve or an outpatient portable drainage device. In our series [14], 33 patients were placed on a Heimlich valve, and 6 patients developed a pneumothorax or subcutaneous emphysema; all patients had an expiratory 5 leak or larger ($P < .0001$). Seventeen patients had leaks that resolved by 1 week, 6 by 2 weeks, and the remaining 9 had their tubes removed without problems. Once home on a valve or an outpatient drainage device, most air leaks will seal in 2 weeks; if not, chest tubes can be safely removed regardless of the size of the leak or the presence of a pneumothorax. Thus the careful use of different chest tube settings as well as the liberal use of outpatient drainage devices all help patients go home on POD 3 or 4, despite the presence of leak or being at high risk to get one [14].

Pain medicine protocols to fast-track patients

Uncontrolled pain can often lengthen hospital stay. The best treatment of pain, as with any postoperative complication, is prevention. The authors have presented several prospective studies on specifics ways to reduce pain [16–19] such as a rib sparing, nerve sparing (via the use of an intercostal muscle flap), muscle-sparing thoracotomy. We also employ a drill to create holes in the inferior rib to avoid the lower intercostal nerve. In addition, the use of pre-emptive analgesia before rib spreading also reduces the pain of thoracotomy [20]. Despite the use of all of these techniques shown by randomized trials to reduce pain and a functional epidural, some patients still complain of severe pain in the hospital, however. Identification of the patients who are at the most risk of having this problem before surgery enables one to help stay on top of the patients' pain issues. Patients who are likely to have pain control issues are those who are chronic users of narcotics, sleeping pills or anti-anxiolytics. Young muscular men are also at risk to have more pain then an elderly thin man or women. Patients who come in to surgery already addicted to medicines will require much higher doses of narcotics to help control their pain and anti-anxiolytics to control their emotions to deal with the postoperative setting. In addition, the authors add several different classes of pain medicines in the immediate postoperative period in addition to the narcotics. We use COX-2 inhibitors as well as nonsteroidal anti-inflammatory drugs, because they are not addictive.

Failure to fast-track: identification of risk factors preoperatively; patient characteristics that portend fast-tracking failure

Several studies have examined potential risk factors for postoperative complications following lung resection. The risk factors consistently identified are elderly age, obesity, preoperative habitual pain medication or anti-anxiolytic use, poor preoperative pulmonary function tests (PFTs), smoking up to the day of pulmonary resection, and pneumonectomy (Table 2) [21–23]. In the authors' recent series evaluating barriers to fast-tracking [24], we found that obese (BMI >38), elderly (>70 years old) age, and those who had poor preoperative pulmonary function (FEV_1 <45%), percent of carbon monoxide diffusing capacity [DL_{CO}] <50%) were often unable to be fast-tracked on our original fast-tracking postoperative algorithm. We then implemented specific changes to this fast-tracking protocol for these select groups of patients and re-evaluated our outcomes.

The changes implemented were as follows: The obese underwent aggressive mobilization and physical therapy, increased aspiration precautions, and the avoidance of continuous positive airway pressure (CPAP) machines at night. In the elderly we avoided the use of narcotics and epidurals. We replaced the preoperative epidural insertion with the intraoperative placement of subpleural pain pumps. Those who had poor PFTs were sent for pulmonary and physical therapy rehabilitation before surgery, and had more frequent respiratory treatments after surgery. Following modification of the fast-tracking algorithm, the length of stay was reduced by the protocol changes from 6.7 to 4.9 days ($P = .024$) in the elderly, from 5.7 to 4.8 days in the obese, and from 6.2 to 4.3 days ($P = .008$) in those who had FEV_1 less than 45%. The morbidity was reduced from 26% to 17% in the elderly ($P = .046$), from 29% to 20% ($P = .027$) in the obese, and from 45% to 23% in those who had an FEV_1 less than 45%. Overall mortality was also reduced 3.9% to 2.1% ($P = .014$) [24].

Table 2
Groups of patients undergoing elective pulmonary resection who often fail fast-tracking and recommendations. Identification and planning preoperatively are key

Patient characteristic	Preoperative	Intra-hospital
Elderly (>70 years old)	Avoid epidural. Ensure social support postoperatively.	Avoid narcotics postoperatively. Avoid sedative medications and narcotics after POD 3.
Obese (BMI >38), especially those with comorbidities (diabetes, sleep apnea, poor mobility)	Preoperative pulmonary rehabilitation Preoperative physical therapy (in patients who have difficulty mobilizing)	Aggressive physical therapy/ambulation Aspiration precautions on POD 1 (keeping head of bed at least 35°, thick liquid diet). No CPAP use
Chronic narcotic, anti-anxiolytic or alcohol users	Preoperative evaluation by anesthesia for pain control regimen	Adjust postoperative pain medication regime to reflect currently used doses. Continue currently used anti-anxiolytics.
Poor preoperative PFTs (FEV_1 <50%)	Preoperative pulmonary and physical rehabilitation Stress importance of smoking cessation as far in advance of surgery as possible	Increased frequency of respiratory treatments

Abbreviation: CPAP, continuous positive airway pressure.

Some previous series have cited elderly age, usually defined as 70 years old or older, as a preoperative risk factor [25]; however, in the authors' recent study assessing the short and long term results of elderly patients who had non-small cell lung cancer (NSCLC) and who underwent lung resection [26], we found that elderly patients had similar morbidity and mortality risk as compared with their younger counterparts. We did find significantly greater likelihood of developing a major morbidity in elderly patients who had a history of neo-adjuvant radio-chemotherapy [26]. Others have found similar results [27,28].

It may be beneficial to discharge elderly patients from the hospital early. Prolonged hospitalization in elderly patients often leads to confusion, "sundowning," and other problems such as nosocomial infections and skin breakdown. Of course patients cannot be discharge unless they are clinically ready and unless they have social support. Elderly patients who live alone or with an elderly spouse, who often has his or her own health issues, should be carefully counseled before discharge. The plans for postoperative convalescence need to be established before pulmonary resection, and this step alone helps reduce fast-tracking failures. The authors set up plans for discharge before surgery. Because a rehabilitation center or a nursing home may be needed for those with unreliable social support at home, plans should be made (insurance coverage, bed availability, etc) before the elective operation. This avoids the failure of fast-tracking for social reasons.

Obesity has been identified as an independent risk factor for surgical site infection, and the obese population has a higher than normal incidence of perioperative deep venous thrombosis, bronchopneumonia, and pulmonary embolism. For these reasons, physicians must make thorough evaluations to properly identify and address medical comorbidities and other issues associated with obese patients such as diabetes, poor nutritional status, immobility, and so forth. The authors advocate aggressive physical therapy, pulmonary toilet, pain control, and aspiration precautions for obese patients. In our own practice we have observed that maintaining aspiration precautions on POD 1, including a thick liquid diet, avoiding use of CPAP following pulmonary resection, and family and patient education for aspiration precaution have significantly reduced morbidity.

Other risk factors such as pneumonectomy, smoking immediately preceding surgery, and history of neo-adjuvant therapy have also been associated with increased morbidity and thus greater likelihood of failing fast-tracking

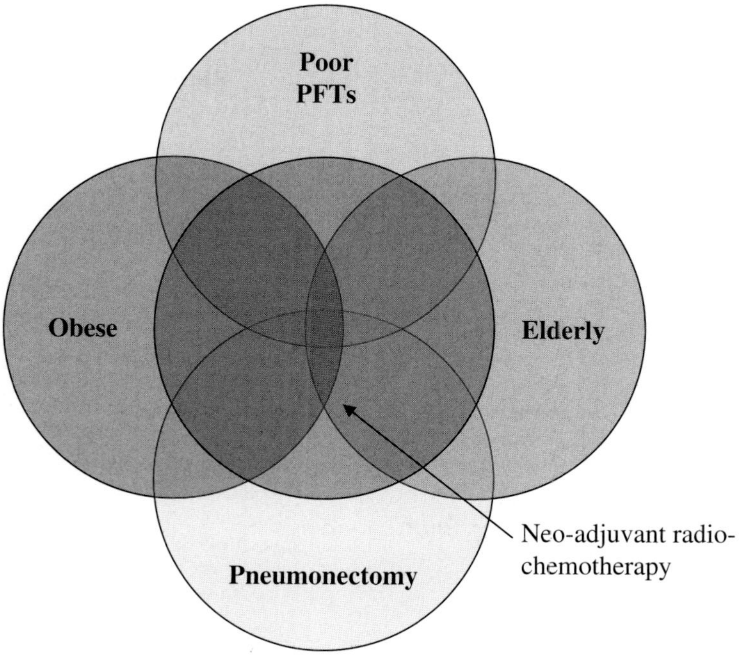

Fig. 1. Diagram of cumulative effect of the individual risk factors for failure to fast-track. The greater the overlap, the greater the risk of failing to fast-track.

protocols [29]. Such risk factors have an additive quality, meaning that the more risk factors patients have, the greater their likelihood of failing to fast-track (Fig. 1).

Summary

Fast-tracking protocols or postoperative care computerized algorithms have been shown to reduce hospital length of stay and reduce costs [2,30]; however, not all patients can be fast-tracked. Certain patient characteristics may put patients at increased risk to fail fast-tracking. Additionally some patients have multiple risk factors that have an additive effect that puts them at an even increased risk to fail fast-tracking (see Fig. 1), and more importantly, to significant morbidity. It is a mistake to force these protocols on all patients because it can lead to increased complications, readmissions, and low patient and family satisfaction. By carefully analyzing surgical results via accurate prospective databases, the types of patients who fail fast-tracking and the reasons they fail can be identified. Once these characteristics are pinpointed, specific changes to the postoperative algorithm can be implemented, and these alterations can lead to improved outcomes. The authors have shown that by using pain pumps instead of epidurals in elderly patients we can improve outcomes and still fast-track octogenarians with minimal morbidity and high-patient satisfaction. We have also shown that the increased use of physical therapy and respiratory treatments (important parts of the care of all patients after pulmonary resection, but a limited resource in most hospitals) may also lead to improved surgical results for those who have low $FEV_1\%$ and $DL_{CO}\%$. Further studies are needed. Although fast-tracking protocols cannot be applied to all, the vast majority of patients who undergo elective pulmonary resection, even those at high risk, can undergo safe, efficient, and cost-saving care via preset postoperative algorithms. When the typical daily events are convened each morning and the planned date of discharge is frequently communicated with the patient and family before surgery and each day in the hospital, most patients can be safely fast-tracked with high satisfaction and outstanding results.

References

[1] Zehr KJ, Dawson PB, Yang SC. Standardized clinical care pathways for major thoracic cases reduce hospital costs. Ann Thorac Surg 1998;65:914–9.

[2] Wright CD, Wain JC, Grillo HC, et al. Pulmonary lobectomy patient care pathway: a model to control cost and maintain quality. Ann Thorac Surg 1997; 64:299–302.

[3] Cerfolio RJ, Pickens A, Bass C, et al. Fast-tracking pulmonary resections. J Thorac Cardiovasc Surg 2001;122:318–24.

[4] Sadovsky R. When to remove a chest tube? A randomized study with subsequent prospective consecutive validation. J Am Coll Surg 2002;195:658–62.

[5] Baumann MH. What size chest tube? What drainage system is ideal? And other chest tube management questions. Curr Opin Pulm Med 2003;9:276–81.

[6] Cerfolio RJ, Bryant AS. Results of a prospective algorithm to remove chest tubes after pulmonary resection with high output. J Thorac Cardiovasc Surg, in press.

[7] Cerfolio RJ. Recent advances in the treatment of air leaks. Curr Opin Pulm Med 2005;11:319–23.

[8] Cerfolio RJ, Bass CS, Katholi CR. Prospective randomized trial compares suction versus water seal for air leaks. Ann Thorac Surg 2001;71:1613–7.

[9] Marshall MB, Deeb ME, Bleier JI, et al. Suction vs water seal after pulmonary resection: a randomized prospective study. Chest 2002;121:831–5.

[10] Cerfolio RJ, Bryant AS, Singh S, et al. The management of chest tubes in patients with a pneumothorax and an air leak after pulmonary resection. Chest 2005;128(2):816–20.

[11] Brunelli A, Sabbatini A, Xiume' F, et al. Alternate suction reduces prolonged air leak after pulmonary lobectomy: a randomized comparison versus water seal. Ann Thorac Surg 2005;80(3):1052–5.

[12] Brunelli A, Monteverde M, Borri A, et al. Comparison of water seal and suction after pulmonary lobectomy: a prospective, randomized trial. Ann Thorac Surg 2004;77(6):1932–7 [discussion: 1937].

[13] Brunelli A, Al Refai M, Monteverde M, et al. Pleural tent after upper lobectomy: a randomized study of efficacy and duration of effect. Ann Thorac Surg 2002;74(6):1958–62.

[14] Cerfolio RJ, Bass CS, Pask AH, et al. Predictors and treatment of persistent air leaks. Ann Thorac Surg 2002;73:1727–30.

[15] Brunelli A, Monteverde M, Borri A, et al. Predictors of prolonged air leak after pulmonary lobectomy. Ann Thorac Surg 2004;77(4):1205–10 [discussion: 1210].

[16] Cerfolio RJ, Bryant AS, Patel B, et al. Intercostal muscle flap reduces the pain of thoracotomy: a prospective randomized trial. J Thorac Cardiovasc Surg 2005;130:987–93.

[17] Cerfolio RJ, Bryant AB, Bass CS, et al. A prospective, double-blinded, randomized trial evaluating the use of preemptive analgesia of the skin before thoracotomy. Ann Thorac Surg 2003;76:1055–8.

[18] Cerfolio RJ, Price T, Bryant AS, et al. Intracostal sutures decrease the pain of thoracotomy. Ann Thorac Surg 2003;76:407–11.

[19] Cerfolio RJ, Bryant AS, Maniscalco LM. A Non-divided intercostal muscle flap further reduces the pain of thoracotomy: a prospective randomized trial. Annals of Thoracic Surgery, in press.

[20] D'Andrilli A, Ibrahim M, Ciccone AM, et al. Intrapleural intercostal nerve block associated with mini-thoracotomy improves pain control after major lung resection. Eur J Cardiothorac Surg 2006;29(5):790–4 [Epub 2006 Feb 14].

[21] DeMaria EJ, Carmody BJ. Perioperative management of special populations: obesity. Surg Clin North Am 2005;85:1283–9.

[22] Kearney DJ, Lee TH, Reilly JJ, et al. Assessment of operative risk in patients undergoing lung resection. Chest 1994;105:753–9.

[23] Linden PA, Bueno R, Colson YL, et al. Lung resection in patients with preoperative FEV1 $< 35\%$ predicted. Chest 2005;127:1984–90.

[24] Bryant AS, Cerfolio RJ. Analysis of surgical results leads to improve post-operative algorithms and fast-tracking of high risk patients after pulmonary resection. in press.

[25] Spaggiari L, Scanagatta P. Surgery of non-small cell lung cancer in the elderly. Curr Opin Oncol 2007;19: 84–91 [review].

[26] Cerfolio RJ, Bryant AS. Survival and outcomes of pulmonary resection for non-small cell lung cancer in the elderly: a nested case-control study. Ann Thorac Surg 2006;082:424–30.

[27] Gridelli C, Maione P, Colantuoni G, et al. Chemotherapy of non-small cell lung cancer in elderly patients. Curr Med Chem 2002;9:1487–95.

[28] Sorenson S, Glimelius B, Nygren P, et al. A systematic overview of chemotherapy effects in non-small cell lung cancer. Acta Oncol 2001;40:327–39.

[29] Ramnath N, Demmy TL, Antun A, et al. Pneumonectomy for bronchogenic carcinoma: analysis of factors predicting survival. Ann Thorac Surg 2007; 83:1831–6.

[30] Lee SC, Tseng HY, Wang KY, et al. Effect of a clinical pathway on selected clinical outcomes of pulmonary lobectomy. Zhonghua Yi Xue Za Zhi (Taipei) 2002;65:7–12.

ELSEVIER
SAUNDERS

Thorac Surg Clin 18 (2008) 119–124

THORACIC
SURGERY
CLINICS

Index

Note: Page numbers of article titles are in **boldface** type.

A

B

C

1547-4127/08/$ - see front matter
doi:10.1016/S1547-4127(08)00020-0

H

I

K

L

P